Vertigo and Dizziness

Professor Jaydip Ray is an ENT Consultant at Sheffield Teaching Hospitals and Professor of Otology/Neurotology at the University of Sheffield and Sheffield Hallam University. He completed his specialist training in Birmingham and undertook fellowships in Cambridge, Australia and the USA.

He is the communications lead for the ENT Clinical Research Network of the National Institute for Health Research. His main research interests include the management of balance disorders, complex hearing loss and implantable hearing solutions. He has been the chief investigator on several multicentre research projects.

Jaydip also plays an active role in teaching and training, and lectures widely at several national and international conferences. He is the Training Programme Director for ENT in Yorkshire and Humber Deanery and is the academic representative for the Specialist Advisory Committee for ENT.

Jaydip is married with two children and enjoys spending time with his family, plus reading, travelling and badminton.

CU00953134

Overcoming Common Problems

Vertigo and Dizziness
Your guide to balance disorders

PROFESSOR JAYDIP RAY

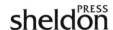

First published in Great Britain in 2018

Sheldon Press
36 Causton Street
London SW1P 4ST
www.sheldonpress.co.uk

British Library Cataloguing-in-Publication Data
A catalogue record for this book is available from the British Library

ISBN 978-1-84709-443-8
eBook ISBN 978-1-84709-444-5

Typeset by Falcon Oast Graphic Art Ltd, www.falcon.uk.com
First printed in Great Britain by Ashford Colour Press
Subsequently digitally reprinted in Great Britain

eBook by Falcon Oast Graphic Art Ltd, www.falcon.uk.com

Produced on paper from sustainable forests

This book is dedicated to my parents,
who have always inspired me to help others

Contents

Acknowledgements

I am most indebted to my family for their unwavering support in all my endeavours. Also to my teachers, trainees and, most importantly, my patients, from whom I continue to learn. My special thanks to David Baguley, Roger Gray, Julie Ward, Pam Shaw, David Throssell, Claire Shepherd and Hayley Skidmore for their continued support and guidance. I would also like to acknowledge the Sheldon team and the immense input of all the contributors, who are:

- **Chapters 1 and 3 – Simon Carr**
  Consultant ENT Surgeon, Sheffield Children's Hospital and Bradford Royal Infirmary
- **Chapter 5 – Panos A. Dimitriadis**
  Academic Clinical Fellow in ENT, Sheffield Teaching Hospitals
- **Chapter 11 – Dev Bhattacharyya**
  Consultant Neurosurgeon, Sheffield Teaching Hospitals
- **Chapter 12 – Dr Jo Sessions**
  Clinical Psychologist, Regional Department of Neurotology, Sheffield Teaching Hospitals
- **Chapter 13 – Christopher Bowse**
  Chief Technical Audiologist, Regional Department of Neurotology

Introduction

The fact that we walk on two legs, unlike the majority of animals, is often taken for granted. What we don't always appreciate, however, is the complexity of the processes that enable us to do this, and the fine alterations the body and brain are constantly making while maintaining our balance and posture. Very often, it's only when things go wrong that we give much thought to the processes involved. This book examines how we keep our balance, how this apparently simple feat interlinks with other organs and systems in the body and the consequences when this delicate and intricate system fails. We look at the vexed question of dizziness, which affects so many people, and explain why a straightforward statement such as, 'I feel dizzy' may actually beg more questions than it answers. Balance disorders cause a great deal of distress and confusion: in the UK, 5 out of every 1,000 people consult their GP each year because of vertigo, while 30 per cent of people report dizziness at some point.

People's vocabulary can be vague and subjective when it comes to describing these symptoms, however. Neither dizziness nor vertigo is a disease as such – rather, both are symptoms. 'Dizziness' in particular tends to be used as a catch-all, general term of reference, which is useful as a starting point but needs to be developed a lot more before it can mean anything medically reliable. We will examine in detail what constitutes dizziness and its unpleasant twin, vertigo, the differences between them and the various conditions they might indicate. Hopefully this will give you a clearer idea of what to tell your doctor if you need to make an appointment. On this point, some people fear that their symptoms indicate a little-known neurological disease that conventional tests fail to pick up. Dizziness and vertigo can indeed be baffling. It's important to realize, though, that they do often involve anxiety, which can affect a person's perception of his or her condition and have an impact on that person's quality of life in a more general way as well. So, this book also looks at psychological strategies to manage balance disorders. The main focus, however, is on physical diseases;

we cover a wide range of balance disorders, including those that are little known and/or have only recently come under close investigation. This book also tells you what medical treatments you might expect for the various conditions, including lifestyle management, medication, implants and surgery. We also look at future research. Armed with all this information, you should, we hope, emerge with a much better understanding of balance disorders, although this book is not a substitute for your own doctor's advice, which you should seek for proper diagnosis and treatment.

Let's start by looking at balance and posture, and the processes by which these remain stable.

1

Balance and posture

Simon Carr

'Balance' is your ability to maintain the centre of gravity of your body within its base of support, whereas 'posture' is defined as the alignment of your body and limbs. There are several types of posture: 'static' (standing, sitting and lying, for example) and 'dynamic' (such as walking, running and lifting). It is during movements that the balance system is under the most strain.

By design, the human body is a rather unstable machine. Due to the fact that two-thirds of our mass is located in the top two-thirds of the body, furthest from the ground, we are in a constant state of instability and, therefore, reliant on a balance system that is constantly assessing information coming in and adjusting our positioning as a result. This is most apparent when an aspect of the balance system fails, making falls more likely.

Maintenance of your posture and balance relies on the inter-action of several different systems, including your eyes (ocular system), inner ears (vestibular system), and joints, especially of your legs (proprioceptive system), which interact to sense the environment. The information from these systems then travels to the balance centre of your brain with messages from your joints travelling via the spinal cord, where it is processed. When it reaches your brain, the information from the different systems is pieced together and an appropriate response of the eyes, muscles and joints is performed, all of which take place in a fraction of a second.

Eyes (ocular system)

The eyes play a major role and vision is arguably the most import-ant sense for maintaining your balance. Your vision is constantly assessing the surrounding environment that you are either stand-ing in or moving on and the nature of objects around you, the information being fed back to the balance centre in your brain.

Inner ears (vestibular system)

The role of your inner ears is to assess movements of your head relative to gravity and the horizon and enable you to keep looking at an object even when your head moves in different directions.

Your inner ears are made up of three semicircular canals and two otolithic (ear stones) organs. The three semicircular canals in each inner ear lie within three different planes: one lateral (horizontal), one posterior (backmost) and one superior (uppermost). They work in pairs: the lateral canals work together and the superior canal works with the opposite posterior canal. The canals are fluid-filled and have an enlarged (ampullated) end, which contains the sense organ (cupula), a jelly-like dome-shaped structure with hair cells protruding into it which are attached to the balance nerve. When you turn your head, the fluid in the canals shifts, which causes the cupula to move, thus moving the hair cells and triggering a signal that travels along the balance nerve. This information is used by your balance centre to tell the brain where the head is positioned in relation to the environment – that is, if the head is tilted or turned to the left or right or looking up or down. This information is used to keep your eyes looking at a particular object when your head is turning and also to enable your eyes to remain stable when your head moves while you are walking or running.

The two otolithic organs are called the saccule and utricle. They are called otolithic organs as they contain small crystals of calcium carbonate. These are embedded into a jelly-like substance with hair cells protruding into it. The saccule detects gravity, whereas the utricle detects horizontal acceleration, such as when you are accelerating in a car. When your body is subjected to vertical acceleration (gravity) or horizontal acceleration (for example, in a car), the gel layer in the organ moves more quickly than the crystals sitting within it, causing the gel layer to distort. This distortion is detected by the hair cells, which triggers a signal that travels down the balance nerve to the brain.

Acting together, the inner ears provide information about the position and movements of your head in relation to what is around you. If you have problems with your inner ears you will be significantly more unsteady in low light conditions, such as when you get out of bed in the night, as your brain will not receive sufficient balance information from your eyes due to the darkness. The only information will come from your joints.

Joints (proprioceptive system)

It is essential for the brain to be aware of the position of your arms and legs, particularly the lower limbs, at any moment in time. If your balance is to be maintained on a variety of terrains, then the brain must be able to interpret what actions are required in order to keep you upright. This information is derived from the signals your joints send to your brain via your spinal cord.

Brain

The information from all of these systems is processed by a particular region of your brain called the cerebellum, which is situated at the back of the brain. The cardiovascular system (heart and blood vessels) plays an important role in maintaining the blood supply to the brain.

What happens when it goes wrong?

Any insult to any part of your balance system will have an effect on your ability to maintain your balance. This can be due to visual problems, such as cataracts, and arthritis, which can affect the proprioceptive system, conditions affecting the vestibular system, such as vestibular neuritis (VN; see Chapter 3), or a problem with the balance centre in the brain, such as chronic alcohol abuse. These systems can also be affected by various medications, such as certain antibiotics (gentamicin, for example) and anti-epileptic medications (such as phenytoin).

If the blood supply to your brain is reduced, you will feel dizzy. The most common cause of this is orthostatic hypotension, which is when the blood pressure doesn't rise quickly enough on sitting or standing up, resulting in momentary dizziness – a head rush. This can happen as part of the ageing process or can be part of certain conditions, such as diabetes.

As the human body ages, the chance of one or several of these systems developing a problem increases. In the UK, falls are the most frequent and serious type of accident in people aged 65 or over, and are the main cause of disability and the leading cause of death from injury in those aged 75 or over. Every year more than 1 in 3 of the population (3.4 million) over 65 have a fall that can cause serious injury and even death. Fractures sustained as a result of falling are increasing and are even more than the number of people having a stroke or heart attack.

2

The impact of balance disorders

The term 'dizziness' is used to describe all manner of balance disorders. The trouble is that balance problems are of various types, differing in onset, duration, severity and frequency. Hence, the impact of each condition will vary and will affect people differently. Remember, dizziness is a subjective symptom that only you can feel. Those around you (even those close to you) may have no idea when you are dizzy and how you might be feeling. It is therefore very useful to share your feelings and experiences with them so that they can appreciate the effect it is having on you.

It is irrefutable that loss of balance has a significant impact on your mobility, confidence and independence. This causes anxiety, stress, depression and may subsequently result in an inability to carry out simple activities of daily living.

The wider impact of dizziness is huge: 30 per cent of the UK population is estimated to experience symptoms of dizziness or imbalance by the age of 65 years and it is the most common reason for visits to a doctor by those aged over 75; 1 in 3 adults in the community has significant dizziness at any given time and up to 14 per cent of people stop work because of imbalance.

Stress can sometimes be both the cause and the effect of dizziness. Stress reactions can be triggered by events in your environment or personal life. The body responds by increasing the release of stress-combating hormones. These are meant to switch on the 'flight, fight or submit' mode and can cause an increase in your heart rate and respiration rate, a heightened state of anxiety and arousal with muscle tension, pain and headaches. The hyperventilation itself can cause dizziness and the muscle tension can cause stiffness and reduced mobility exaggerating the dizzy symptoms. This feeds the cycle of anxiety, tiredness, low mood and depression, which then leads to altered behaviour aimed at avoiding activities that bring on the dizzy symptoms. This behaviour can affect your immediate social environment, work or personal relationships.

The common features to look out for are:

- rapid heartbeat
- rapid breathing
- muscle tension
- tightness of the chest
- restlessness
- irritability

- sleep disturbance
- constant tiredness
- loss of interest
- loss of self-confidence
- social withdrawal.

You will already be aware that one of the biggest risks arising from balance disorders is of a fall. Falls in people over 65 years are a leading cause of confinement and death and are termed as one of the 'giants of geriatrics'.

The social, occupational and economic costs of balance disorders to the individual, society and health services are profound, resulting in repeated medical attendances and costly investigations.

One of the most common features related to dizziness and falls is a 'fear of falling'. This is a well-known consequence. It sets up a downward spiral of negative thought processes, compounding the problem further as the person curtails various daily activities, which leads to reduced mobility and physical fitness that, unfortunately, further increase the risk of falls and injuries. This also leads to reduced social interaction, depression, isolation resulting in loss of activity, earning and productivity. As we live longer, keeping active and preventing falls is a huge challenge to society.

People with neuro-disability (the impairments an individual can experience following a traumatic brain injury or stroke) also have significant posture, balance and stability issues. Your doctor will usually arrange for a rehabilitation plan through a falls service. This will usually include exploring the history of falls and an assessment of gait, balance, mobility, muscle weakness, osteoporosis risk and functional ability.

If you have a balance disorder, then you will be at a high risk of falling. The risk is hugely increased if you have comorbidities (two or more coexisting medical conditions that are additional to an initial diagnosis) and take lots of medications.

People aged 65 and older have the highest risk of falling, with 30 per cent of people older than 65 and 50 per cent of people older than 80 falling at least once per year. Older women with diabetes (especially those with neuropathy – damage to nerves causing numbness or weakness) have a higher risk of falls and hip fractures.

The human cost of falling to the individual includes distress, pain, injury, loss of confidence and independence, as well as the effects on relatives and carers. According to the National Patient Safety Agency, the healthcare cost for treating falls in England and Wales is estimated to be in excess of £15 million per year. This figure rises to an estimated £2.3 billion per year, however, when associated costs, such as fracture management and long-term care provision, are taken into consideration. Fragility fracture management alone (for any fall from a standing height or less that results in a fracture) is estimated to cost the NHS about £1.7 billion per year, and the major determinant of this cost is length of hospital stay.

Dealing with the problem

Given the implications of dizziness, it is important to have a clear understanding of the background problems and their causation. The next few chapters will help you explore some of these issues in a systematic fashion.

The first step in self-help is relaxation and to adopt fall prevention strategies. Regular exercise to maintain your core strength, stability and mobility is proven to be very beneficial. Making sure your glasses are checked regularly and a healthy diet (especially vitamin D) will help. If you experience dizziness and instability, an uncluttered environment free of trip hazards will help to prevent injuries. Other areas to address are footwear and lighting.

Dizziness and its related problems set up automatic reactions that are linked to negative thoughts. As previously discussed, there is a combination of anxiety, depression, anger and guilt.

Other problems are rumination, avoidance and denial. Here you end up going round and round in circles thinking about the dizziness itself and the impact it has on you instead of focusing your energy on addressing measures that might help resolve the problem. This reduces your motivation to engage in solutions and keeps you perpetually in your current state. It also pushes you to avoid all movement and become less and less mobile. There is some evidence that mindfulness and cognitive behaviour therapy might help you to understand your condition better and motivate you to engage with the rehabilitation strategies.

It is important to remember that some balance disorders (as you will see shortly) may be chronic. While a quick-fix cure may not exist yet for the majority of conditions, a lot can be achieved by self-help strategies, motivation and long-term engagement with therapy to control the symptoms.

One useful strategy might be to take charge of your own health and well-being, address the problems as they arise, have realistic expectations and recognize your limits. In some cases, reasonable adjustments to your work, social and family environments may be necessary. Never assume that everyone understands all the problems the dizziness is causing you. Indeed, there may be many that are invisible to others . It always helps to explain clearly how you feel and how your condition might affect you and your performance, either regularly or sporadically. That gives you and the people around you the mutual understanding and respect, space and commitment to make adjustments to fit in with the condition and its effects.

You will see in the following pages that a lot of the management strategies are simple and intuitive. They are not obvious, however, to those who have never experienced balance problems or seen them in others. The importance of self-education and motivation cannot be overemphasized, to enable both you and the people around you to appreciate the problem and act in a supportive and constructive way to minimize its impact on the day-to-day quality of life.

3

Common conditions

Simon Carr and Jaydip Ray

The symptoms of balance disorders can occur in a number of different ways and the experience of them differs between individuals. It is, therefore, important for your clinician and you to confirm that you are both speaking about the same sensation. If you ask someone to describe his or her dizziness, you are likely to get one or more of the following responses:

- vertigo
- spinning sensation
- confusion, disorientation
- lightheadedness
- muzzy head
- spaced out feeling
- difficulty concentrating
- headache or migraine
- intolerance of motion or motion sickness
- imbalance or unsteadiness
- walking on cotton wool
- tumbling down feeling
- nausea or vomiting
- visual disturbance.

There are certain symptoms that are more likely to be associated with the inner ear balance system than with other parts of the system. Vertigo is an hallucinatory sensation of rotation, either of your surroundings around you or rotation of you within your surroundings. You may feel as though objects tip to one side or that you are being pulled or pushed to one side or another. Dizziness may only occur when you are in certain positions, such as when you are rolling over in bed or looking up or down.

Let us now examine some of the most common balance conditions and how they may affect people.

Disorders of the inner ear (vestibular) system

Benign paroxysmal positional vertigo

Benign paroxysmal positional vertigo (BPPV) is one of the most common disorders of the inner ear and can be caused by an upper airway viral infection or following whiplash or a head injury. 'Benign' means that it is not cancerous, 'paroxysmal' means recurrent sudden episodes of symptoms and 'positional' means that the symptoms are triggered by certain movements of the head. 'Vertigo' is dizziness with a sensation of movement – you feel as if the world is moving around you or that you are moving when you aren't. Often you will also feel sick.

The link between vertigo occurring in certain positions and abnormal eye movements was first noticed and highlighted by Robert Bárány in 1921. As described earlier, in Chapter 1, there are two otolithic organs in the inner ear balance detector: the saccule, which detects gravity – that is, vertical movement – and the utricle, which detects horizontal movement. Both of these organs have a jelly-like layer with crystals of calcium carbonate embedded within it. If these crystals detach from the jelly-like layer of the utricle they can float off down the semicircular canals. Due to where it is located, the posterior (backmost) semicircular canal is most commonly affected by gravity. When you roll over on to either your right or left side (depending on which side is affected) or look up or bend forwards, the canal is stimulated. This results in vertigo after a slight time delay, which lasts for seconds to minutes and then eases.

There are two theories as to why this occurs: canalolithiasis and cupulolithiasis. Canalolithiasis was first described by John Epley, who theorized that the crystals detached from the utricle and became free-floating in the posterior semicircular canal. When your head is moved to a certain position, the free particles initially move with the inner ear fluid, but then sink in the fluid due to gravity. This movement stimulates the movement detector in the semicircular canal (the cupula) producing a spinning sensation or vertigo. The eyes exhibit a typical short-lasting twisting movement (nystagmus) directed towards the lowermost part of the ear. In cupulolithiasis, first described by Harold Schucknecht, the crystals become stuck to the cupula, which makes it heavier and

more unstable. This causes vertigo that lasts for longer than canalolithiasis.

In order to find out if this is the cause of your dizziness, the
doctor will perform a Dix-Hallpike test. They will ask you to sit on
an examination couch and then lie back quickly with your head
over the end of the couch, tilted about 30 degrees towards the floor.
The good side is usually tested first and then the side on which
the symptoms are present is tested. A typical positive response results in vertigo, which starts after a time delay and lasts for seconds
to minutes before easing off. When you sit up again, the vertigo
will go the other way for a few seconds before stopping. The doctor
will see a rolling of the eyes towards the floor, which will speed up
and then slow down. On sitting up again, the eyes will roll in the
opposite direction. If the diagnosis is confirmed, then the doctor
will perform a particle repositioning manoeuvre, such as the Epley
manoeuvre. This involves lying in a series of different positions to
move the crystals from the semicircular canal to their original position in the utricle. As this is being performed, you may feel further
bouts of vertigo and, as you sit up for the last part, you may feel a
dropping sensation as the crystals relocate to the utricle.

Approximately 85 per cent of people will require a treatment
of one Epley manoeuvre. Occasionally, people may require repeat
manoeuvres. There is a small subgroup of people who do not respond to the Epley manoeuvre. This group may require surgery to
close off the semicircular canal to prevent the movement of crystals
and fluid within it.

You may also be able to administer the Epley manoeuvre at
home, with caution and some help. The exact method is shown in
videos on the internet (see, for example, <www.primarycareshef-
field.org.uk/cases/ent>).

Vestibular neuritis

Together with BPPV, VN is one of the most common types of dizziness related to the inner ears. It usually occurs following a viral
infection, such as a cold or flu, which spreads from the upper
respiratory tract (the nose and nasal cavity, the pharynx and the
larynx) to the inner ears. This may affect the balance organ alone,
which is known as VN, or together with the hearing organ, the
cochlea, which is known as acute labyrinthitis.

VN results in severe vertigo, usually with vomiting, which may last for several days. After the initial acute, severe phase, the symptoms, although they may still be present, tend to lessen in severity. If you experience these symptoms, the doctor may give you a medication called prochlorperazine, which can be administered by mouth, under the tongue or else injected, in severe cases. This acts as a vestibular sedative, which means that it dampens down the messages from the inner ear to the balance centre of the brain, which can help to relieve the vertigo and vomiting. In addition to this, it is important that you maintain your fluid intake as vomiting can cause dehydration. Occasionally, if it is very severe, you may need to be admitted to hospital.

The natural history of the condition is that the balance centre of your brain shuts down the messages from the balance organ of the side that is affected, which reduces the severity of the symptoms. Over time, your brain undergoes 'compensation', which means that the brain slowly reintroduces the messages from the previously affected balance organ. The timescale of this phase can vary greatly, taking up to several months. During this recovery phase you may have episodes of 'decompensation', when you may feel off balance. This may occur when you are travelling on an escalator in a busy shopping centre, for example. The combination of movement, bright fluorescent lights, people moving around you in different directions and loud noise can overstimulate the balance system, causing a sense of imbalance. It is important to stress, however, that this should not put you off stimulating the balance system as recovery may be delayed if it is not exercised. If you do not recover, you may benefit from balance rehabilitation therapy.

Ménière's disease
Historical background

This enigmatic and often disabling condition was originally described by a French physician, Prosper Ménière, who published a series of articles in Paris in 1861, describing the characteristics of the condition that we now call Ménière's disease (MD).

Ménière was the first to link the episodes of vertigo to the inner ear balance organs. He described the typical relapsing and remitting episodes of spinning sensation or rotatory vertigo along with hearing loss, ringing in the ears (tinnitus) and nausea and vomiting.

He also noted the sudden drop attacks (falls without loss of consciousness) in some of those affected and background low-level poor balance as the condition progressed. Various other symptoms have also been suggested as being linked with the condition, including hearing fluctuating, fullness of the ears and an exaggerated feeling of loudness (termed 'loudness recruitment').

How is it caused?

MD is an enigmatic condition and there are still many unanswered questions about its causation. MD is thought to be caused by an excess amount of fluid within the inner ear, known as endolymphatic hydrops, which was first shown in 1938 by Hallpike and Cairns who reported their findings from dissection of the temporal bones (the part of the skull that houses the inner ear hearing and balance organs) of those with documented MD. They demonstrated swelling of inner ear fluid (endolymphatic fluid) and spaces with distortion of the inner ear membranes (Reissner's membrane). There are people who have endolymphatic hydrops who do not develop the classic symptoms of MD, however, so the exact mechanism by which this excess fluid causes MD is still not fully understood.

Symptoms

MD consists of episodes of vertigo that can last for several hours and be associated with vomiting and photophobia (light hurting the eyes). People often report having to go to bed during these episodes. Just before the start of the episode of vertigo, you may experience ringing (tinnitus) and a feeling of pressure (aural fullness) in one ear, which can act as a warning (aura) of the imminent onset of vertigo. Typically, you would also have a fluctuating inner ear hearing loss. At the start of MD the hearing of low frequency sounds is usually affected, but as the disease progresses, the hearing loss may become permanent and affect all frequencies.

MD can occur at any age, but usually does so during the late thirties to mid sixties with more people in the older age group being affected than the younger. The number of new cases each year ranges from between 4 and 28 per 100,000 of the population and the number of established cases ranges from 50 to 513 per 100,000 of the population.

The American Academy of Otolaryngology (1995) developed diagnostic criteria in 1972 to help with the diagnosis of MD. There have since been several revisions and Table 1 shows the current criteria.

Table 1 Criteria for diagnosis of Ménière's disease

Diagnosis	Criteria
Certain MD	• Definite MD as below and confirmation by tests.
Definite MD	• Two episodes of vertigo lasting longer than 20 minutes. Documented hearing loss on at least one occasion.
	• Tinnitus and/or fullness of the ear.
	• All other causes excluded.
Probable MD	• One episode of vertigo lasting longer than 20 minutes. Documented hearing loss on at least one occasion.
	• Tinnitus and/or fullness of the ear.
	• All other causes excluded.
Possible MD	• Episodic vertigo of Ménière's type without documented hearing loss.
	• All other causes excluded.

Will it get worse?

Attacks may resolve of their own accord or MD may progress to the 'burnt-out' stage, whereby the attacks will stop, but there will be no residual balance activity or hearing in the affected inner ear. The timescale for this is variable and can take decades. The other problem is that up to 50 per cent of those affected may develop the disease in both ears. This can result in people losing all inner ear balance function and in bobbing oscillopsia, which is when the eyes cannot fix on an object or the horizon when walking, causing the eyes to 'bob' up and down with each footstep, leading to significant difficulty in maintaining balance and posture. This may be in addition to severe inner ear hearing loss on both sides – a truly disabling condition indeed.

Your doctor may request balance testing, which can help in the diagnosis of the condition and also determine the functionality of the inner ear balance system, not only in the ear that is affected, but also in the unaffected ear, which is important if the affected ear is going to be treated surgically.

Treatment

The good news about this disabling condition is that there are various treatment options available. While they may not cure the condition, there is a high chance of achieving control of the symptoms. Treatment options are addressed in a step-wise manner. Initially, simple changes to your lifestyle and diet may be all that is required to control mild symptoms. Medicines may be used to control further symptoms or prevent larger attacks. When simple measures fail, your doctor may recommend surgical treatments, which are described in some detail later on in this chapter. These steps are described below and summarized in Table 2 on page 18.

Lifestyle   Lifestyle changes are aimed at reducing the collection of fluid inside the inner ear and avoiding triggers. These triggers, such as salt, caffeine, chocolate or red wine, can increase the vertigo and avoidance of these is widely practised. Restriction of salt in the diet has also been the cornerstone of treatment for more than half a century. This is based on the idea that reduction in salt lowers the amount of fluid load present in the body, which in turn reduces fluid in the inner ear. While there is no convincing evidence to either support or disprove this idea, many people report some relief of their symptoms with this regime and, hence, this is still widely advised by many specialists. Most regimes suggest taking less than 2 g of sodium per day but a more liberal practical approach, with more allowance of sodium per day, would work just as well. The suggested association of Ménière's symptoms with caffeine, chocolate and red wine is harder to explain. All these are known triggers for migraine as well, and the parallel association between Ménière's and migraine may be the best-fit explanation so far. If lifestyle measures don't help control your symptoms, medical treatment may need to be added.

Medicines   Betahistine (sold as Serc) works by improving the blood flow around the inner ear to reduce the amount of fluid within it. The evidence for this is weak, but the treatment is widely used, due to patients reporting benefits. Cinnarizine works by reducing the blood pressure in the blood vessels around the inner ear, which reduces the amount of inner ear fluid. It also works by blocking other receptors that are linked to sickness and nausea, thus reducing these symptoms. This helps to make it a useful medication in vertigo, MD and motion sickness.

Diuretics (water tablets), such as bendroflumethiazide, may be recommended in an attempt to reduce the blood pressure around the inner ear, reducing the inner ear fluid. Prochlorperazine (sold as Stemetil) is an anti-sickness drug, which blocks signals from the inner ear to the balance and the vomiting centres in the brain. This is a useful medication to take when you feel the onset of an attack is imminent as it can lessen the severity of it and also control the associated vomiting.

Grommet If the symptoms persist in spite of maximal medical therapy, then surgery would be the next treatment option. Usually, this would start with the placement of a grommet (ventilation tube) in the eardrum of the affected side. The grommet works by enabling pressure equalization either side of the eardrum, which can help if your main symptom is fullness or pressure in the ear.

Additional equipment Pulse pressure therapy using the Meniett® device in conjunction with a grommet is of uncertain benefit. This has a probe, which fits into the ear canal and delivers air down the ear canal, increasing the ear pressure, travelling through the grommet and increasing the pressure in the middle and inner ear. Some have reported that they find this beneficial for treating episodes of vertigo.

Middle ear medications Intratympanic (in the middle ear, through the ear drum) injections of a steroid, such as dexamethasone, can be performed under local anaesthetic in the outpatient clinic to reduce any inflammation in the inner ear. It can prove very useful for an acute episode or a period of increased frequency of attacks and has the added benefit that it does not have a negative effect on the hearing. The treatment can be repeated and also topped up using steroid-based ear drops through a grommet. There are various routes for delivering medications through the eardrum. The simplest method is delivering it by injection through an anaesthetized eardrum using a fine needle. This can be repeated as needed.

Another method is the Silverstein wick, which is placed in contact with the round window (one of the entry points to the inner ear) and anchored to the eardrum with a grommet, through which it protrudes into the ear canal. Any eardrops in the ear canal are absorbed by the wick and transported to the round window and into the inner ear. The grommet keeps access open, allowing drops to be delivered over a certain time period. A more recently introduced product, which is currently under investigation, is steroid medication in a gel . This allows for a continuous slow release of the medication to the inner ear.

The choice of intratympanic medication has gone through various phases, from the use of gentamicin (an antibiotic) alone to a combination of gentamicin and steroid and then to steroid alone.

If the attacks are severe and your hearing is poor, then a chemical labyrinthectomy using gentamicin might be offered. The gentamicin is delivered via an intratympanic injection. This can be performed under either local or general anaesthetic. Gentamicin is an antibiotic that is toxic to the inner ear balance organ in certain concentrations, a side effect which can be utilized to treat this condition. It usually affects the cells of the balance organ, but can affect the hearing as well. Therefore, it is usually offered to those whose hearing has been affected significantly by MD, but some people are so severely affected by vertigo that they are willing to risk their hearing in order to treat it. Occasionally, this treatment needs to be repeated to achieve complete control of vertigo. A recent study demonstrated, however, that steroids used on their own were as effective as gentamicin in reducing the number of attacks and, therefore, current practice is steadily shifting towards the use of steroids.

Surgery If the previous treatments fail, then more radical surgical options may be needed. Some surgeons would offer surgery on the endolymphatic sac – a non-sensory organ of the inner ear that is thought to regulate the formation of fluid. Opening this sac and placing a small drain in it reduces the amount of inner ear fluid, thereby reducing the vertigo. The advantage of this procedure is that the hearing can be preserved.

In severe cases a surgical labyrinthectomy can be performed, which involves removing all three semicircular canals of the inner ear balance system. As the end organ is removed, the fluctuating and

Table 2 Summary of treatment options for Ménière's disease

Lifestyle modification	Medication	Surgery
• Low-salt diet. • Avoid triggers – caffeine, chocolate and red wine.	• Betahistine. • Cinnarizine. • Bendroflumethiazide. • Prochlorperazine for acute vertigo episodes.	• Grommet (ventilation tube) and/or Meniett® device. • Intratympanic steroid injections. • Chemical labyrinthectomy – intratympanic gentamicin. • Endolymphatic sac surgery. • Surgical labyrinthectomy. • Vestibular nerve section.

debilitating symptoms of MD are eliminated. There is a trade-off, however, with permanent loss of balance function on the operated side. The balance apparatus of the opposite side slowly compensates for this loss to regain equilibrium.

A more recent surgical development is plugging of the three semicircular canals to stop them functioning, thereby reducing their ability to cause attacks. The experience with this technique is very small, however, so there is need for more operations to be performed and the effects monitored before it will be widely accepted as the main surgical option.

Cutting the balance nerve so that the abnormal signal from the balance organ is not passed on to the balance centre of the brain is a procedure that used to be performed more readily, but the results were variable.

John the HGV driver

John was a delivery truck driver with a wife and two young children. He started getting occasional attacks of vertigo with nausea and vomiting at the age of 41 years. Initially these were diagnosed as labyrinthitis and treated symptomatically. The frequency, duration and intensity all increased over the next three years and he had attacks without warning. He was referred to the neurotology department at the hospital and was diagnosed with unilateral MD. He had to give up driving due to the uncontrolled attacks of vertigo and made a voluntary declaration to the DVLA. The specialist and his GP supported him to be redeployed to an office job with the same employer.

Initially the treatment was with lifestyle and dietary modifications, and medications in the form of betahistine and a low-dose diuretic. His symptoms worsened so he underwent the insertion of a grommet with instillation of steroid in the middle ear. This controlled his symptoms very well and his quality of life improved. After two years, however, his symptoms recurred, so the treatment was repeated. He has now been symptom free for more than six years. To rehabilitate his hearing, he was fitted with a hearing aid.

Migraine

Recently, the awareness and understanding of migraine has improved. Migraine, however, is complex and we still don't fully understand the mechanism by which it causes vertigo. There is a great deal of crossover between MD and migraine (see also vestibular migraine in Chapter 4). Similar to MD, migraine tends to cause vertigo, which can last for several hours and sometimes be associated with vomiting and photophobia (sensitivity to light). You may have, or previously have had, migraine or there may be a strong family history of the condition. You may have features of classical migraine with vertigo, including headache and visual symptoms such as zigzag lines or flashing lights. The diagnosis requires that at least 50 per cent of these episodes are associated with a headache, but it doesn't always need to be the predominant symptom. Vestibular migraine doesn't usually affect hearing, which aids in the differentiation of this condition from MD.

Medical management is the mainstay of treatment. Lifestyle modification consists of avoiding triggers, as in MD. If you experience migraine, you will usually know what triggers these attacks. Simple analgesia, such as paracetamol or ibuprofen, can be helpful in treating the attacks, even if there is no associated headache, as the pathways that cause a headache migraine are similar to those that cause the vertigo migraine. A step up from this would be medications to help prevent the attacks occurring, such as amitriptyline, propranolol or topiramate. These are discussed in greater detail in Chapter 4.

Link between MD and migraine

In a joint project studying the link between MD and migraine, two neurotology groups from Sheffield and Sydney reported three significant findings.

- A family history of MD (33 per cent) or migraine (21 per cent) is more common in MD patients – that is, someone with MD is more likely to have a close relative who has MD or migraine than someone who doesn't have MD.
- A history of migrainous headaches is more common in patients with MD (45.1 per cent) than those who don't have MD.
- Those with a past history or a family history of MD or migraine have a higher likelihood of being diagnosed with MD than those who don't have such a background.

Brenda

Brenda was 36 years old when she experienced recurrent episodes of vertigo. These were unprovoked and lasted for a variable time period, from 2 to 30 hours. There were no associated hearing symptoms, although Brenda experienced significant nausea and abdominal cramps. During an attack, she was intolerant of bright light and sound, which caused her to retreat to a dark, quiet room until the attack passed. After it had passed, Brenda was left with what she described as a 'muzzy head' for many days. There were some dietary triggers, such as excess coffee. There was also a strong family history of migraine.

Brenda worked for a construction company and, due to difficulties coping with computer screens and working in an open-plan office, she was finding it increasingly hard to work. Repeated absences due to the attacks were viewed with less and less sympathy by her employers.

The results of all the clinical tests were essentially normal. A working diagnosis of MD was made and treatment started. As this failed to help her symptoms, Brenda was also advised on strategies to cope with visually provoked vertigo and given related exercises to practise. Unfortunately this caused her symptoms to worsen and by this time she was finding it impossible to carry on with her job. She saw another consultant and the diagnosis of vestibular migraine was considered. Relevant dietary modifications and lifestyle measures were advised, in addition to daily amitriptyline (10 mg per day). To her relief, there was a dramatic improvement in her symptoms. Brenda was able to continue with her job successfully and has now been promoted to a management position.

4

Other conditions

In recent years, light has been thrown on a number of conditions that were less well known previously.

Vertebrobasilar infarcts

There has been increasing awareness about the link between circulatory problems and balance disorders. The main blood supply to your brain comes from two sources: the anterior (front) circulation from the carotid arteries (the large blood vessels on either side of your neck) and the posterior (back) circulation from the vertebral arteries (the large arteries that arise in the vertebral column at the back of your neck). The two systems join to form the Circle of Willis in the middle of your brain. The posterior circulation is crucial for your balance system as it supplies the balance centres in the brainstem and the cerebellum (responsible for coordination of movement). Sudden vestibular episodes with other neurological symptoms should arouse suspicion of associated problems in the posterior circulation in the brain, the symptoms of which can be:

- visual disturbance
- numbness of face or extremities
- confusion/loss of consciousness/clumsiness
- weakness of legs/ataxia (problems with walking)
- difficulty swallowing (dysphagia)
- problems with speech (dysarthria/dysphonia)
- focal neurological symptoms (impairments that affect a specific region of the body), either with loss of sensation or power.

In contrast to a pure vestibular (inner ear) balance problem, a vertebrobasilar ischaemic drop attack is often described as a sudden lower extremity weakness – 'My knees felt like they were buckling and giving way under me.' The following facts are worth noting.

- It is known that 20 per cent of mini strokes – transient ischaemic attacks (TIAs) – and larger ones – cerebrovascular accidents (CVAs) – are from the vertebrobasilar system, which is the main feeder for the posterior circulation.
- The symptoms of TIAs of the vertebrobasilar circulation may be either vertigo or deafness on its own. Of the two symptoms, vertigo is the most common initial isolated symptom of decreased blood flow through the posterior circulation (five times more common with associated neurology). The classic syndrome associated with a problem relating to the blood supply in the cerebellar artery distribution (an artery that provides blood to the cerebellum) is called the lateral medullary syndrome or Wallenberg syndrome. The symptoms can be diverse. Here you may experience vertigo, severe balance disorders, nausea, vomiting, facial numbness, facial weakness, difficulty swallowing and articulating speech sounds and a wider sensory loss on the opposite side of the body.
- It is also well established that you are at higher risk of a stroke after a TIA arising from the vertebrobasilar system than a TIA arising from the carotid artery. You also have a higher incidence of repeated stroke in this situation.
- It is well known that if you have a high incidence of stroke risk factors, such as high blood pressure, diabetes, raised cholesterol, obesity, smoking and high alcohol intake, you are likely to have a decreased blood supply to the vertebrobasilar area. The need for awareness of this problem cannot be overemphasized and you would be advised to reduce the modifiable risk factors – stress, smoking, alcohol, cholesterol – with dietary advice and lifestyle modifications.

Graham

Graham, a 75-year-old man, had a history of repeated spells of spinning sensation of sudden onset over the last nine months, often associated with nausea, vomiting, alteration in hearing, blurring of vision, tingling and numbness of the same side of the face and a weak feeling in the lower limbs that recovered each time. There had been six such episodes in the last three months. Graham's grandson, who lived close by, recalled him having three similar but milder episodes over a two-year period about four years ago. He had high blood pressure, high alcohol intake and had smoked 20 cigarettes a day for over 50 years. He had been prescribed prochlorperazine for the last six months without any improvement of his symptoms. A full neurotological (elements of the ear that relate to the brain) examination yielded no notable results, but his hearing tests showed high-frequency hearing losses on both sides in keeping with age-related hearing loss (presbycusis). Magnetic resonance angiography (scans that provide an image of your blood vessels) showed significant differences in posterior circulation between the two sides. A further neurological consultation was undertaken. The prochlorperazine was stopped and risk factor reduction measures were put in place, along with the introduction of statins (medication to lower cholesterol) and anti-clotting medication. Despite this, Graham went on to have a mild stroke within the next six months, but made a full recovery.

This illustrates the importance of awareness in the medical community so that early preventative measures can be put in place before further damage is done. The risk of unwarranted long-term use of so-called 'balance medication' in the absence of a clear diagnosis needs to be emphasized. These not only have no benefit in these situations but can also add to the problem as a result of their own side effects.

Vestibular migraine

This is another balance disorder where the cause and management have remained elusive for a very long time. Many patients have been wrongly diagnosed and treated inappropriately. The problem lies in the symptoms often resembling those of other balance conditions, such as MD (discussed in Chapter 3). Many authors have highlighted the link between balance symptoms and migraine for many years, but it is only recently that the condition has been recognized as an independent entity and treated as such.

It is now thought to be one of the most common causes of vertigo and spontaneous episodic vertigo. More people with migraine have vertigo than those with tension-type headache. 'Vestibular migraine' is the accepted term for migraine that has primarily vestibular symptoms, such as vision disturbance, hearing changes and dizziness. The other names commonly used to describe this condition are migraine-associated vertigo, migrainous vertigo and migraine-related vestibulopathy. The vertigo in these situations can range from dizziness brought on by head movement or position to ataxia (lack of coordination when walking) of variable duration.

How is migrainous vertigo caused?

The cause is not as yet clearly understood, although various theories have been put forward. One suggests that there is a release of certain chemicals in your brain called neuropeptide mediators (substance P) or serotonin (5HT). There are several well-established theories on the source of the migrainous symptoms themselves, including the concept of spreading depression of the cortex (superficial surface of the brain) where a wave of nerve excitement spreads through the cortex-releasing chemicals (called neurotransmitters) that give rise to the classic aura followed by a throbbing headache and that of neurovascular instability. In this, an initial constriction of the blood vessels causing the aura is followed by a rebound dilatation of the blood vessels resulting in the throbbing pain. It is thought that vestibular migraine may also be due to a combination of both these phenomena, together with an associated or accompanying excitation of the central and peripheral vestibular sensors resulting in the feeling of imbalance.

As a result of the above confusion, clear diagnostic criteria have been set up by the International Headache Society to help develop uniformity in diagnosis and reporting of vestibular migraine. The most accepted classification and diagnostic criteria divides it into two main categories: definite and possible vestibular migraine. It might be worth gaining an understanding of this classification (see Table 3).

There are a few additional features of the condition. For example, females are three times more likely to suffer from this condition than males. The other most commonly associated features include:

- rotational vertigo
- intolerance of head movement/visual stimuli
- positional vertigo.

It is important to recognize that the episodes of vertigo may occur even without migrainous headaches in 6 per cent of cases. The distribution is as follows:

- **always** 45 per cent
- **sometimes** 48 per cent
- **never** 6 per cent.

Table 3 Classification of vestibular migraine

Definite vestibular migraine	Possible vestibular migraine
• Episodic vestibular symptoms of moderate severity.	• Episodic vestibular symptoms of moderate severity.
• Either:	• One of the following:
– a current or previous migraine;	– a current or previous migraine;
– at least two episodes of migrainous vertigo with migrainous headache, photophobia, phonophobia (sound sensitivity), aura.	– a migraine during vestibular episodes;
	– migraine precipitants of vertigo;
	– response to migraine medication.
• Other causes excluded.	• Other causes excluded.

Who will I see?

Usually you will see your GP, an ear, nose and throat (ENT) specialist or neurologist. All of them will rely on an accurate medical history to arrive at the diagnosis.

What tests are available?

There are as yet no specific diagnostic tests for vestibular migraine. A detailed history in line with the diagnostic criteria is the key to arriving at a firm diagnosis.

Your doctor may still order some tests to exclude other balance conditions and to establish the presence of other concomitant conditions. There is also a range of magnetic resonance imaging (MRI) scans that can exclude the presence of any abnormalities or growths in the intracranial hearing and balance pathway.

Triggers

You will normally be very aware of the common triggers that set your symptoms off:

- **dietary** caffeine, chocolate, alcohol, especially red wine and port, aged cheese
- **activity** exertion, dehydration, sleep deprivation, periods, bright light
- **weather** barometric changes, seasons.

Other conditions that need to be differentiated

The diagnostic confusion between MD and migraine is often problematic to many practitioners as both have episodic vertigo, hearing loss and tinnitus as symptoms. The key differentiators are that the vertigo in vestibular migraine can last a lot longer than in MD – more than one day – and is more likely to be associated with phonophobia (sound sensitivity) and photophobia (light sensitivity). You are more likely to have progressive hearing loss in MD, while this is less likely in vestibular migraine. You are also more likely to have a past history or family history of migraine in both conditions.

'Vertebrobasilar insufficiency' is a reduction in blood supply from the arteries that supply the posterior part of the brain and 'benign paroxysmal vertigo of childhood' (BPVC) is a type of migraine occurring only in childhood.

How to manage vestibular migraine

The management of vestibular migraine is aimed at various levels of severity. The mainstay of treatment is: clear explanation, education and the adoption of lifestyle measures. A clear understanding of the nature of your condition and the main triggers is most useful. If this fails to control your symptoms adequately, you may need additional medication.

The following is a brief overview of the management strategy.

Diary

You will be encouraged to maintain a detailed dietary log over time to link the symptoms to potential triggers through direct association.

Lifestyle

Awareness of the potential role of lifestyle modifications goes a long way towards promoting better control of symptoms and preventing many of the episodes. Indeed, it is key to understand the association between your symptoms and the well-known triggers. Behavioural and dietary modifications may enable much greater control to be achieved of early symptoms. Further, association between anxiety states and migraine and MD has also been proposed and the term 'migraine–anxiety dizziness' (MARD) may help some more anxious patients to understand and deal with their situation more effectively.

Rehabilitation

You may benefit from vestibular rehabilitation if you have problems maintaining stability due to persistent background imbalance.

Medical

The medical treatments are divided broadly into two categories: those preventing the occurrence of the symptoms (prophylactics) and those curtailing the symptoms when they occur (abortives).

Prophylactics

These are used to reduce the likelihood of migrainous attacks and are usually used individually rather than in combination:

- anticonvulsants (topiramate)
- beta blockers (propranolol)
- calcium channel blockers (verapamil)
- tricyclic antidepressants (amitriptyline).

Abortives

These medications can stop or significantly shorten the duration of the attacks. Simple analgesics can be helpful, but the main medications in this category are the triptans, such as sumatriptan. These work alongside the neurotransmitter serotonin and are effective in treating migraine.

Newer treatments

Other treatments that have been tried include nerve decompression, neuromodulation and botulinum toxin injections.

Victoria

Victoria, a 41-year-old schoolteacher, started having symptoms of prolonged unsteadiness lasting for about two days at a time. These episodes were preceded by a variable period of feeling 'spaced out' and intolerance of daily sounds, making it very difficult to function in a noisy primary school. After a day or so she would develop a vice-like headache on top of the imbalance. Usual over-the-counter medications were ineffective. She was referred to the neurotology department at the hospital as she was starting to have problems at her workplace due to repeated absences. The results of her examination were normal and the hearing thresholds were within normal limits. A provisional diagnosis of vestibular migraine was made and an explanation of possible triggers and relievers was provided, along with instructions to keep a detailed diary of diet, balance episodes and possible triggers. This exercise revealed a clear association between excess daily coffee consumption and work-related stresses from late-night working preparing teaching plans and reports leading to overexertion. Simple dietary and lifestyle modification, as well as a low dose of amitriptyline, rapidly resolved all her symptoms.

Superior semicircular canal dehiscence

Superior semicircular canal dehiscence (also called SSCD or Minor's syndrome after Lloyd Minor, who described this condition in 1995) is thought to be caused by an anatomical abnormality in the temporal bone that houses the semicircular canals which form the inner ear balance apparatus. As mentioned earlier, we have three pairs of semicircular canals (lateral or horizontal, posterior and superior) that are roughly at right angles to each other. They monitor angular motion in their respective planes. The balance apparatus is housed in one of the hardest bones in our body called the otic capsule. The hardness of the bone is to prevent any external disturbances influencing it. If the bony covering over the superior semicircular canal is missing, due to an anatomical defect, then your balance apparatus is not protected from some external stimuli. This results in direct communication between your superior semicircular canal and your intracranial compartment, which houses the brain and the brain fluid (called cerebrospinal fluid or CSF). Dizziness results from changes in sound and pressure. The sudden eye movements (called nystagmus) that occur as a response to this are in the plane of the superior semicircular canal. Similarly, minor changes in pressure in the intracranial compartment can also be transmitted to the balance apparatus, which results in the conglomeration of symptoms that you may experience when there are minor changes in your environment.

The common symptoms all have interesting names. Here are descriptions of them.

Autophony

In this situation you might be able to hear an internal echo of your own voice when speaking and also hear internal bodily noises, such as eye movements, jaw joints, chewing, neck movements, own footsteps.

Tulio phenomenon

Here you might be intolerant of loud noise and sudden noises, which may bring on attacks of nausea and/or vertigo.

Bobbing oscillopsia

You may experience an uncontrolled bobbing of the visual scene whenever you move, such as when you are a passenger in a car going over a hump.

Pulse-synchronous oscillopsia

Internal pulsations may create a disruption of the visual scene which may bob up and down as a result.

Hyperacusis

You might become intolerant of loud noises or even day-to-day sounds, resulting in a very unpleasant sensation from sounds. These may include the sound of a hairdryer or a vacuum cleaner or even cutlery and plates (McKenna et al., 2010).

Balance symptoms

These range from varying degrees of dizziness, rotatory vertigo or spinning attacks or a sense of chronic disequilibrium.

Low-frequency conductive hearing loss

The majority experience a low-frequency hearing loss, which makes it difficult to understand speech at times.

Fullness in the affected ear

You may have a sensation of pressure and fullness. This may, in turn, cause you undue anxiety about the possibility of having some sinister disease, such as a tumour lurking in the background. You are unlikely to have the other symptoms of a brain tumour or any other such condition, however. A scan can exclude this possibility quite easily.

Pulsatile tinnitus

You might hear a pulsatile noise synchronous with your heartbeat that is difficult to switch off or ignore (McKenna et al., 2010).

Fatigue

All or some of the symptoms above often cause significant stress and anxiety, resulting in a feeling of being fatigued all the time.

Headache/migraine

This is also an associated symptom as the headaches may be directly related to the condition.

Other causes that need to be differentiated

Some of the symptoms may mimic otosclerosis (a condition of abnormal bone deposition in and around the otic capsule), MD, labyrinthitis and BPPV.

Are there any tests for it?

The cornerstone of diagnosis is a very high index of suspicion in relation to the symptoms listed above. The main objective tests are high-resolution computerized tomography scans (HRCT). Your doctor will usually request these special scans and have them reported on by an experienced neuroradiologist (a radiologist specializing in brain imaging). It is easy to miss the condition unless the scans are reformatted and viewed in the appropriate plane.

The other objective test that is becoming popular is the cervical vestibular evoked myogenic potential (cVEMP – see Chapter 9) measurement. This test records the contraction of the neck muscles in response to sound impulses. Normally the traces in the test level off at a sound intensity of around 85–90 dB, but in this condition an abnormally low threshold of about 60–70 dB is noticed.

How is this condition managed?

The condition can be very debilitating due to an intolerance of day-to-day sounds and pressure changes. This, combined with the occasional delay in diagnosis until you see the appropriate specialist, can be very frustrating and affect your social and professional life. Therefore, a high index of suspicion is required and appropriate investigations need to be ordered early to confirm or exclude the diagnosis.

Once a firm diagnosis has been established, you may choose to manage it conservatively, with lifestyle adjustments, or have surgery. The surgical options can be very rewarding in most instances and include either covering (resurfacing) the dehiscent portion of the superior canal or plugging the two limbs of the canal (canal plugging) from behind the ear and mastoid bone (part of the skull located behind the ear). The main risks of surgery are possible hearing loss and only a partial resolution of the symptoms.

Steven

Steven, a 45-year-old man, started getting symptoms of unsteadiness, vertigo, nausea, bobbing oscillopsia (bouncy vision), tinnitus and intolerance of daily sounds. These started mildly with appearance of additional symptoms over two years.

He was given prochlorperazine in primary care without much benefit. Subsequently, he noticed that he could hear internal body noises in quiet settings and got a very strong feeling of vertigo on straining. He was then given antidepressants and referred to a neurologist and then on for neurosurgery.

A CT scan showed a developmental anomaly (a small brain protrusion called a Chiari malformation, previously known as an Arnold-Chiari malformation), for which he had a routine neurosurgical procedure. His balance symptoms continued to become more noticeable over the following two years and he had to stop work and driving. At this point he was referred to the neurotology department at the hospital.

An HRCT scan with reformatting confirmed a diagnosis of SSCD on both sides. Further confirmation was obtained by non-suppression of large waveforms down to 70 dB on vestibular evoked myogenic potential (VEMP – see Chapter 9) measurement. The diagnosis was discussed with Steven and he was given appropriate information and directed to relevant websites to help him come to an informed decision on management strategies. After considering all his options, he decided to undergo plugging of both limbs of the superior semicircular canal sequentially with a 12-month gap between the two procedures.

The majority of his balance symptoms resolved with surgery, albeit with a slight but manageable drop in his hearing. He had already had advice and support for his tinnitus and continued to keep the strategies in place after the operations. He managed to return to his original job and to driving.

Steven's case demonstrates how rare or newly recognized conditions can be missed unless the specialist is considering them in the differential diagnosis and requesting the right investigations.

Bethany

Bethany was self-employed and owned three high street shops. She had experienced occasional mild, short-lasting unsteadiness on straining and noticed that she could hear internal bodily noises, such as eyeballs moving and neck muscles creaking. Around the age of 32 years, she started experiencing additional symptoms: tinnitus, mild hearing loss, problems focusing after sudden movements, echoing of her own voice and footsteps. The latter symptom made her very concerned and she slowly closed her businesses and became housebound as she felt she was being followed by someone when she would hear footsteps on a dark evening. She was treated with increasing doses of antidepressants on the presumed diagnosis of factitious functional disorders. She was referred for secondary care and diagnosed with unilateral SSCD after extensive testing and imaging. The surgical treatment involved plugging of the two limbs of the offending superior semicircular canal via the mastoid bone behind the ear canal. This resolved most of her symptoms with preservation of her hearing and balance.

Other rarer conditions

Cervicogenic vertigo

This is a controversial condition. Although you may experience balance symptoms with neck movements, it is unusual to find specific abnormalities to account for these balance symptoms. Sometimes there might be a history of neck injury or of neck symptoms with a background of degenerative changes due to ageing or arthritis. You might experience a combination of either episodic balance problems associated with specific neck positions or a more persistent vague, 'floaty' feeling modulated with neck movements. There may also be significant neck stiffness, neck pain and limitation of neck movements.

The old theory of reduction in blood supply to the posterior (vertebrobasilar) circulation of the brain during neck movement is vigorously disputed. In this theory, it was suggested that kinking of your vertebral artery brought on by neck movement resulted in reduced blood flow to your balance organ. This was thought to produce the momentary balance symptoms that are relieved by resuming a neutral neck position. Although this is a very attractive explanation and is still widely used, it is too simple to be true. The counter argument is that the vertebrobasilar artery is the main blood supply to the posterior circulation of the brain. Any kinking of such a major artery should give you a conglomeration of multiple neurological symptoms rather than just some imbalance alone. While this debate continues, the real cause remains elusive.

Physical examination usually finds nothing remarkable, apart from some tension in the neck muscles without any specific neurotological symptoms. Lying and standing blood pressure measurements are useful. Diagnostic vestibular tests usually return normal results. It is, however, useful to do a carotid Doppler test to check for any narrowing of the carotid arteries.

The mainstay of management of this condition is physical therapy to free up neck movements, with physiotherapy exercises and improving mobility.

Vestibular paroxysmia

In this rare condition you might experience a sudden severe episode, as if you had an abrupt 'push' or a 'shove' from the side. This comes without warning, is momentary and unpredictable and can sometimes result in the person dropping to the floor without any loss of consciousness.

Physical examination may find nothing remarkable. Hyperventilation may produce a slow nystagmus (rhythmic eye movements). High-quality MRI scans may demonstrate a loop of blood vessel that is irritating the balance nerve. Medical treatment with carbamazepine may help in some cases. Surgical intervention involving microvascular decompression may be helpful in conjunction with neurosurgery where a vascular loop can be seen clearly on the MRI scan.

Bilateral vestibulopathy

This is a condition where there is loss of function in the balance apparatus on both sides. It is somewhat akin to a twin-engine plane losing power in both engines and, hence, is extremely debilitating. Fortunately, this is not very common. It occurs mostly from unknown causes, but can be the result of progressive autoimmune ear disease, bilateral MD or taking systemic ototoxic medication (medicines that damage the inner ear, hearing and balance organs), such as gentamicin.

As mentioned, this condition is very disabling for those who experience it. All complain of dizziness and bobbing oscillopsia (bobbing of the horizon) with difficulty maintaining balance and walking normally in the dark. Those unlucky enough to lose normal functioning of both balance organs tend to walk with a wider than normal gait and may need additional support, such as a walking stick or an umbrella, for stability. It is difficult to perform tandem gait tests (walking in a straight line with one foot in front of the other, a bit like a roadside test to see if a driver is over the limit) with eyes closed and there is a tendency to fall over. Caloric responses (involuntary reflex eye movements in response to irrigation of the external ear canal with warm and cold water) and vestibular evoked myogenic responses (muscle response to a loud click or tone that can be measured from the eye or neck muscles) may both be absent (see Chapter 9). Rotation chair testing is most useful.

Physical therapy can help. It is also very important to implement fall prevention strategies. Local specialist physiotherapists and falls services can provide support and advice tailored to your situation. In the future, vestibular implants may bring some resolution to this very disabling situation.

Mal de débarquement syndrome

This literally means a feeling of motion continuing after the cessation of movement of a form of transport or having disembarked from a mode of transport, usually a boat or ship. Although this is usually apparent after sea travel, it can also occur after any form of travel. It can affect people differently and can last for a variable period of time.

This has been well recognized for many years and many sailors report this to be a normal part of their lives. It can, however, become clinically disabling in a small minority of people, whether they have been travelling or not. It is unclear what the exact cause of this symptom is and there is debate as to whether it is vestibular or central in origin.

The usual management strategy involves appropriate balance investigations to exclude other conditions and customized balance rehabilitation for desensitization (see Chapter 13 for more details).

> ### Louise
>
> A 31-year-old occupational therapist, Louise had a sensation of persistent movement after returning from a holiday that involved an overnight North Sea crossing on a ferry in rough seas. She continued to feel as if she was 'at sea' for a week after returning. She was given anti-sickness tablets and prochlorperazine by her GP. She was then referred to a specialist when her symptoms failed to settle down after two weeks.
>
> A full medical history and examination showed no specific vestibular deficit and a diagnosis of Mal de débarquement syndrome was made. Louise was helped by desensitization with slow oscillations on the rotatory chair synchronous with her sway, followed by continued desensitization on a virtual reality gaming console for the next two weeks.

CANVAS syndrome

Cerebellar ataxia, neuropathy and vestibular areflexia (CANVAS) syndrome is a rare association between lack of coordination, peripheral nerve damage and loss of balance function. Only a small number of cases have been reported so far and more are needed to develop a clearer picture of the association between these symptoms.

Autoimmune inner ear disease

You might consider this as a diagnosis if there is a rapid progression of hearing loss in both ears. You may have also experienced fluctuating hearing loss, a feeling of fullness in the ears and tinnitus, thus mimicking MD.

Fortunately, autoimmune inner ear disease (AIED) is a relatively rare cause of dizziness, often with hearing loss, and can be associated with connective tissue disorders affecting multiple systems. A number of conditions connected with small blood vessel changes can be associated with balance symptoms.

Typically, the hearing loss in AIED responds to treatment with oral steroid medications, which is not the case for MD. Your doctor may also arrange for an assessment of connective tissue antibodies in addition to vestibular function tests and imaging. The condition is treated with short courses of oral steroids, which can be repeated in cases of exacerbation. The role of immunosuppression using cyclophosphamide is not well established.

Elizabeth

Elizabeth, aged 46, had a history of recurrent vertigo and fluctuating hearing loss. This was initially diagnosed as MD and treated in the usual fashion, but without any benefit. The diagnosis was later revised to vestibular migraine and treated as such, also without benefit. She started developing joint pains, stiffness and dry mouth and eyes. At this point, she was referred jointly to the neurotology and rheumatology departments at the hospital. A diagnosis of AIED with a background of Sjögren's syndrome (a disease in which the moisture-producing glands are affected) was made and she responded very well to low doses of steroids.

Perilymphatic fistula

Perilymphatic fistula (PLF) is described as a suspected leak of the inner ear fluid (called perilymph), due to some defect at the junction of the middle ear and inner ear structures. This can result simply from traumatic or surgical disruption of the oval or round window (the only natural connection between the sealed inner ear and middle ear). It is, however, highly controversial as to whether you might have a spontaneous PLF from congenital weakness in these regions. In this case, you may experience fluctuating hearing loss and fluctuating vertigo. There is also a risk of profound deafness and recurrent meningitis, due to the spread of infection from the middle ear into the brain fluid through the fistula (the passageway).

You may think that the suspected leak should be easy to spot, but a definitive diagnosis by directly inspecting the area with a microscope or endoscope is not always possible, due to the complex layout of the middle ear. The fact that the symptoms occur soon after some trauma to the middle or inner ear, however, provides circumstantial evidence that supports a diagnosis of PLF.

Treatment is usually in the form of bed rest, elevating the head and avoiding straining, as well as treatment of the symptoms of vertigo. If the symptoms persist and there is a strong suspicion of a PLF based on circumstances, the ENT surgeon may be able to explore the middle ear and seal both oval and round windows to close the leak.

Psychogenic vertigo or anxious hyperventilation

This is often seen in people who are prone to severe anxiety and hyperventilation. Taking a careful medical history to discover if there have been any instances of periodic hyperventilation with rapid shallow breathing, palpitations, sweating and anxiety followed by a period of imbalance is useful. Arriving at a diagnosis of this condition is, however, a matter of excluding other possibilities. That is, all other treatable conditions have to be considered and excluded first.

You may test this out by voluntarily breathing rapidly for a few minutes. The rapid shallow breaths wash out the residual carbon dioxide in the lungs and make you dizzy. The dizziness will settle with steady deep breaths. In extreme situations you may need to breathe in and out into a paper bag to restore the carbon dioxide content. A clear understanding and supportive environment are most useful in coping with the symptoms. Anxiolytics (drugs to relieve anxiety) may also be prescribed if necessary.

Some neurological conditions

Atypical Parkinson's disease

Parkinson's disease may initially become noticeable atypically as a movement disorder with balance-related symptoms. Similarly, the symptoms of conditions such as progressive supranuclear palsy and multiple systemic atrophy may also be reported as balance disorders early on. They can also readily be misdiagnosed as Parkinson's disease.

Look out for unsteadiness and a tendency to fall backwards. It may be difficult to go downstairs initially. Mobility will diminish fairly rapidly and there is a risk of becoming wheelchair bound in a few years from the initial onset of symptoms. There may also be difficulty in swallowing that progresses relentlessly and may result in aspiration and infections.

The resting tremor of Parkinson's may not be a symptom, but subtle increased stiffness in the neck and body muscles may become noticeable. Cognitive slowing leading to dementia is also known.

Various strategies may be employed to manage the condition. Parkinson's medications, such as levodopa, may also be tried in some with limited benefit.

Spinocerebellar ataxia (type 1, 2 and 3)

This is a rare inherited genetic condition that surfaces in people from their thirties to their fifties. It commonly involves the coordinating centre in the cerebellum and parts of the spinal cord. There are progressive problems with movement or gait disorder (ataxia), together with other neurological signs related to the long motor nerves in the spinal cord. Treatment is mainly by means of supportive strategies.

Episodic ataxia (type 1 and 2)

This is another rare inherited neurological disorder that is genetic in nature. The first type occurs in infancy, while the second type does not appear until people are in their twenties. The symptoms are episodic ataxias (abnormal walking patterns) with vertigo, nausea, vomiting and cerebellar signs, including lack of coordination and rhythmic jerky movements of the eyes (pendular nystagmus). Episodes of these symptoms occurring may be spontaneous or brought on by physical stress and can last several hours. Treatment mainly takes the form of supportive approaches, although some have reported benefit from taking the drugs acetazolamide and carbamazepine.

5

Balance issues in older people

Panos A. Dimitriadis and Jaydip Ray

The ability of an individual to maintain posture and balance when still (static) and when moving (dynamic) is essential for safe, independent living. Disorders of gait (walking patterns) are common in older people and incidence increases with age. It is estimated that 30 per cent of the UK population experience symptoms of dizziness or imbalance by the age of 65 years and it is the most common reason for visits to a doctor by patients aged over 75. Also, 1 in 4 adults have significant dizziness at any given time. You are likely to be able to name at least two acquaintances who have experienced dizziness in the last six months. Up to 14 per cent of people stop work because of balance problems. The social, occupational and economic costs of balance disorders to the individual, society and health services are profound, resulting in repeated visits to doctors and specialists and costly investigations. The most significant implication is that, if you have a balance problem, you are prone to falls with varying consequences from a simple bruise to a fracture to a fatal bleed on the brain.

Falls

The statistics for falls are staggering: globally, up to 35 per cent of people aged over 65 years fall each year, they are the leading cause of accidental death in people aged over 65 years and there is a 66 per cent chance of having another fall within a year of the first fall. This sets off a spiraling cascade of adverse effects for the individual, including fear of falling, reduced mobility, anxiety, depression and isolation, increased risk of falling and further injuries that can all independently or jointly lead to increased ill health and an increased risk of premature death. According to Age UK, in 2010, one in three older people in the UK had a fall, costing the NHS £4.6 million per day. These figures highlight the substantial financial expenditure and significant pressure on healthcare services that falls cause. Further, they are likely to continue to rise when we take into account the rapid growth of an ageing population.

As discussed earlier, the ability to maintain our posture is the result of a central integration of a number of different inputs from our vestibular organs (inner ear balance apparatus), visual system (eyes) and sensory nerves. This information is analysed and processed in different parts of the brain in an amazingly short period of time and instructions are given to various muscles and organs, resulting in the ability to maintain our balance in different situations, from walking down the street to skiing down the slopes! The fine-tuned coordination of these various structures is essential and malfunctions in any of these can affect our ability to maintain our balance.

Balance problems can be divided into three main categories:

1 feedback problems affecting the transfer of information from the periphery to the brain;
2 execution problems that affect the central integration of the information in the brain;
3 support diseases that impair our ability to perform the instructions given by the brain.

Figure 1 summarizes the different systems involved in maintaining posture.

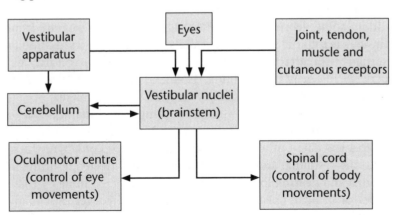

Figure 1 Vestibular sensory input

Suffice to say, as we grow old, a combination of the factors mentioned previously is often encountered. The term 'presbystasis' has been proposed to describe poor balance due to ageing alone. It is similar to 'presbycusis', used to describe poor hearing due to ageing. Sometimes both go hand in hand and need to be addressed proactively to overcome the disabilities caused by them. The management of these problems depends on their nature and is beyond the scope of this chapter, however.

Feedback

Vestibular system (inner ear balance organs)

Any problem affecting your vestibular system can manifest as imbalance, vertigo, instability and insecure gait. Our peripheral balance apparatus, or the vestibular organs, are located in the inner ear and consist of five organs that sense head movement in any direction: the three loop-shaped semicircular canals that detect angular acceleration, the utricle that senses horizontal acceleration and the saccule that senses vertical acceleration. With ageing, there is a decline in the number of cells in these organs as well as the number of nerve fibres of the inferior and superior vestibular nerves that transmit information on head position from the peripheral vestibular system to the brain.

BPPV is a common cause of dizziness. Indeed, 50 per cent of all the cases of dizziness in older people are due to BPPV. In this condition, some debris (crystals of calcium carbonate) migrate from the utricle into the semicircular canals and can cause a sensation of vertigo with certain head movements. For example, you may experience momentary disabling dizziness, lasting a few seconds, when you roll over in bed or tip your head back to look up.

Vestibular neuritis is a disorder resulting from inflammation of the vestibular nerve causing sudden onset of dizziness that can last up to a few days but without hearing loss. In cases of labyrinthitis, both the vestibular and the acoustic nerves are affected resulting in vertigo and hearing loss. Elderly people are affected more by these types of balance episodes and take longer to recover over many months.

CVAs and TIAs are also more common in the elderly than in

younger people. In these situations, the blood supply to the inner ear may be reduced, giving rise to symptoms like those of laby-rinthitis. A careful assessment, especially by a neurologist, is required so as not to miss any major problems that might masquerade as an isolated balance problem.

Bilateral vestibular hypofunction is the reduction or loss of ves-tibular function in both of your inner ear balance organs. Various causes have been suggested, such as ototoxicity (medicines that damage inner ear hearing and balance organs), meningitis and se-quential VN. Sometimes, however, no underlying cause is found and it is attributed to ageing alone and to a reduction in the number of vestibular hair cells. In a recent study, about 60 per cent of people with bilateral vestibular loss reported having a fall.

MD is an inner ear disorder that affects 1 in 1,000 people in the UK. It usually starts at younger ages, but can persist in old age as well. Typically you will experience fluctuating hearing loss, a sensa-tion of fullness and buzzing in the ear (tinnitus), as well as attacks of vertigo that can last up to a few hours. The cause of MD is not clearly understood, but is thought to be related to increased pressure of the fluid in the inner ear (endolymphatic hydrops). Periods of relief in between attacks may vary from days to months. Over time, the ver-tigo attacks may be less severe, but a more permanent sensation of imbalance may develop. Usually this disease affects one ear only, but about 50 per cent of individuals may develop this condition in the other ear as well. It is described in further detail in Chapter 3.

Visual system

Vision plays an important role in keeping the body upright, but the ways in which visual cues are integrated into the balance control mechanism is not fully understood yet. Some epidemiological stud-ies have shown that problems with vision are an independent and significant risk factor for falls. You might have experienced being off-balance when walking in the dark or with your eyes closed. We rely more on our vision to maintain our balance at such times, particularly in cases where the somatosensory and/or vestibular systems are disrupted. Moreover, vision is used to assess the envi-ronment we are in, check for any obstacles or changes in terrain, evaluate the height of steps or stairs and enable safe travel within it. Optical flow provides information about body sway from front to back whereas information from eye movements contains information about side-to-side body sway. Central and peripheral vision are both important for assessing optical flow and are therefore essential in balance control.

The following conditions affecting vision, which are often encountered in older people, can impair the ability to maintain balance (static or dynamic).

Cataracts

A cataract is a clouding of the lens in the eye, which is commonly seen in older adults and causes blurred vision. It is the cause of more than half of the cases of blindness and 33 per cent of visual impairment worldwide.

Diabetes, hypertension, smoking tobacco, alcohol intake and prolonged exposure to direct sunlight are all risk factors for developing cataracts. In some people, lens proteins change, causing the lens to lose its clarity.

Glaucoma

Glaucoma is the second leading cause of blindness in developed countries and is primarily seen in older adults. It represents a group of eye diseases that lead to progressive optic nerve problems and visual field loss. Peripheral vision is initially affected, followed by central vision loss and then blindness if left untreated.

Age-related macular degeneration

Age-related macular degeneration (AMD) is an eye condition in which a small area of the retina, called the macula, is affected and leads to partial loss of central vision. People over the age of 65 are most commonly affected.

The risks of developing the condition are greater if you are female, smoke and are exposed to sunlight for prolonged periods of time, although some individuals have a genetic predisposition to developing AMD.

An undercorrected refractive error

An undercorrected refractive error (blurred vision due to astigmatism, long or short sight) is one of the leading causes of treatable visual impairment.

Presbyopia

Presbyopia is a condition caused by loss of elasticity of the lens, whereby objects that are located near the eye appear blurry.

Eye movement disorders

Nystagmus, other involuntary eye movements, gaze deviations and those caused by lesions in the brain may lead to poor balance.

Somatosensory system and proprioception

The somatosensory system (touch, joints, gravity) receives sensory inputs from receptors throughout the body that indicate the position and movement of the feet, legs, arms, torso and head. This system contributes to our postural stability and any malfunctions of the system can lead to imbalance and increased risk of falling. A recent study that used computerized dynamic posturography (a clinical assessment technique used to quantify balance) suggested that individuals, especially older adults, rely predominantly on proprioception (perception of the position and movement of the body) rather than their vision, to maintain their balance when they are in a light environment with a solid base of support.

Information about the velocity and length of contraction of the muscles is relayed to the nervous system by the muscle spindles, which are stretch-sensitive mechanoreceptors. As a result, appropriate voluntary and reflexive movements are initiated centrally. Some studies have shown that the structure and function of muscle spindles alter as we age. This was observed either in isolation or with associated reduction of local nerve supply. Joint position sense (JPS) and joint motion sense are other commonly used measures of proprioception and their functions have also been found to deteriorate with age.

Another group of receptors that are affected by ageing are the cutaneous receptors. These serve the purpose of nerves in hairless skin. Although they are not considered to be proprioceptors (receptors that signal information to the brain about movement), their function supplements the JPS and movements, and influences muscle activity in the lower extremities by communicating directly with proprioceptors. Vibratory sensation, such as plantar surface (foot sole) vibration, as well as tactile acuity and discriminative touch (two-point sensation) are also affected as we age.

For the different messages to be transferred centrally, a healthy conductive system is required. Human and animal studies have shown that with ageing there is a reduction in the number and density of myelinated peripheral nerve fibres as well as sensory nerve action potential. Apart from ageing, peripheral nervous system disorders such as diabetic neuropathy, hereditary motor and sensory neuropathies and nerve compression syndromes can affect the conduction of tactile and proprioceptive (touch and pressure sensation) information to the brain.

Execution

The brain

Numerous interactions between various parts of our nervous system are necessary for maintaining posture and balance. All levels of our nervous system are needed in the start-up and maintenance of rhythmic stepping and balance, and the ability to adapt to the changing environment. Problems with any of these are likely to lead to poor gait and loss of stability. As mentioned, efficient gait involves more than just our ability to walk. To get from A to B you make a conscious decision as to what route to take, how to interact with the environment and which obstacles to avoid, as well as understanding your physical abilities in conjunction with normal mental function or cognition. For example, wandering is a common feature of people with dementia. When cognition declines, some or all of the levels of the nervous system can be affected, leading to an increased risk of falling.

Different parts of the brain and central nervous system contribute to your balance maintenance strategy. Although slightly technical, let us briefly explore some of these to give you an appreciation of how complex, yet delicate and finely tuned, the system is (see Figure 2).

Frontal lobe

Located at the very front of your brain, the frontal lobe carries out the higher mental processes, such as thinking, decision making and planning. It controls gait and coordinates automatic and voluntary movements. Chronically poor blood supply (ischaemia) in the brain due to disease in the smaller blood vessels commonly

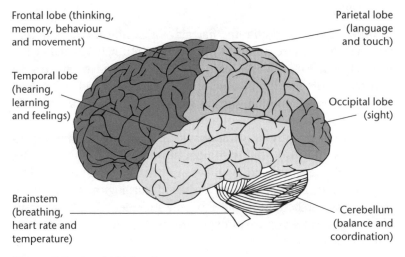

Frontal lobe (thinking, memory, behaviour and movement)

Parietal lobe (language and touch)

Temporal lobe (hearing, learning and feelings)

Occipital lobe (sight)

Brainstem (breathing, heart rate and temperature)

Cerebellum (balance and coordination)

Figure 2 Parts of the brain

leads to changes in the white matter of the brain. Recent studies have shown that higher volumes of white matter lesions are associated with balance, gait and mobility impairments.

Basal ganglia (or basal nuclei)

These structures are strongly connected to the cerebral cortex, brainstem and thalamus. They are located deep inside the base of your brain and are associated with control of your voluntary motor movement, routine behaviours and cognition.

The main components of basal ganglia are the dorsal and ventral striatum, substantia nigra, ventral pallidum, globus pallidus and subthalamic nucleus.

Two movement disorders – Parkinson's disease and Huntington's disease – have been studied extensively. Parkinson's disease results from significant loss of the cells that release dopamine in the substantia nigra and is characterized by a gradual loss of the ability to initiate movement. Its incidence is about 20 cases per 100,000 people and it commonly begins between the ages of 40 and 70. Huntington's disease involves loss of medium spiny neurons in the striatum and is characterized by an inability to prevent parts of the body moving unintentionally. Its incidence is 10 cases per 100,000 people and usually appears in middle age.

Cerebellum

Another region of the brain that plays a significant role in controlling your fine movements (motor control). It is located at the back of your brain, underneath the cerebral hemispheres (like a hair bun). It is like the conductor of an orchestra and is involved in automated locomotion, such as while running, accurate timing, precision and coordination of movement.

Cerebellar atrophy (wasting away) due to ageing or other degenerative disorders is linked with poor movement and increased risk of falls. With ageing there is an average loss of cerebellum Purkinje cells of about 2.5 per cent per decade. Neurological disorders affecting the cerebellum in older people include multiple sclerosis, cerebellar strokes and toxin exposure, such as heavy metals, lithium and phenytoin.

Spinal cord

The spinal cord maintains the rhythm in your stride and is involved in automated locomotion. It sends out nerves to supply segments of your body and muscle groups responsible for movement of different joints.

Support

Musculoskeletal system

Two common features of an aged musculoskeletal system include decline in bone mineral density (osteoporosis) and muscle mass (sarcopenia).

Osteoporosis

Over 3 million people in the UK are affected by osteoporosis, which is often diagnosed following a fracture resulting from a low-impact injury. Hormonal changes after menopause in women, low levels of physical activity, reduction in dietary protein, deficiency of vitamin D or calcium, heavy drinking and smoking and, interestingly, a low body mass index can all contribute to osteoporosis. Individuals with reduced muscle mass and strength are more prone to falling and sustaining a fracture due to poor bone quality.

Kyphosis (hunchback)

A curvature of the spine that causes the top of the back to appear more rounded than normal in the elderly resulting from weakened back extensor muscles. This change in posture shifts the weight of the body forwards and, in turn, affects balance and increases the risk of falling.

Cervical spondylosis

This is a 'wear and tear' degeneration of the vertebrae and intervertebral discs in the neck. It is common, affecting 90 per cent of people over the age of 60 to different degrees. You should suspect this if you are experiencing a combination of neck pain and stiffness, a sensation of 'pins and needles' in your arms or legs and, more rarely, loss of coordination and difficulty walking.

Lumbar spine stenosis

Another age-related change of the spine that can cause you to experience leg pain at rest (sciatica), leg pain with walking (claudication) and tingling, weakness or numbness that radiates from the lower back into the buttocks and legs.

Osteoarthritis

A common condition affecting mainly individuals over 50 years of age. It is a degenerative joint disease characterized by progressive loss of joint cartilage, formation of bony spurs (osteophytes) at the edge of the joints and thickened, inflamed synovium (inner layer of the joint capsule that produces synovial or joint fluid). Besides ageing, risk factors for osteoarthritis include being female, obesity, previous joint injury or disease and genetic factors. You will likely have either a friend or relative with osteoarthritis, complaining of knee, hip and back pain (arthralgia), joint stiffness and swelling. Mobilization and physical activity are decreased due to pain and discomfort, which results in deconditioning, muscle wasting and increased risk of falling.

Gout

A form of arthritis that causes sudden, severe attacks of pain, redness and swelling in the affected joints. It affects 2 per cent of people in the UK and is more common in men than women. Age at onset is usually 30 years for men and after menopause for women. It results from abnormal deposits of sodium urate crystals around the joint cartilage and their release in the synovial fluid. As with other joint and podiatric problems, gout affects normal posture and mobility and predisposes those who have it to falls.

Cardiovascular system

Some studies have linked cardiovascular disease with balance insta-bility and falls that are either associated with loss of consciousness (syncope) or without loss of consciousness. Syncope is defined as a transient, self-limited loss of consciousness with an inability to retain postural tone, which is followed by spontaneous recovery. In the majority of cases, lightheadedness, vertigo or prior faintness precede syncopal episodes. A number of causes have been identi-fied, but the ones most commonly seen are orthostatic hypotension (drop in blood pressure due to change in posture or on standing), carotid hypersensitivity syndrome, neuro-cardiogenic syncope and bradycardia (heart rate under 60 beats per minute).

With non-syncopal falls, an extreme drop in blood pressure when standing up (orthostatic hypotension) has been found by different studies to be an independent risk factor for loss of postural stability and falls. It occurs if you experience a drop of ≥20 mm Hg in sys-tolic or ≥10 mm Hg in diastolic blood pressure after three minutes of standing from lying. Its frequency in people over the age of 60 years has been found to be up to 30 per cent, but it is not always symptomatic. A number of causes have been linked to orthostatic hypotension, including dehydration, medications such as vasodi-lators or diuretics, cardiac abnormalities such as myocarditis and aortic stenosis. A strong association has also been found between postprandial hypotension, which is an excessive decrease in blood pressure following a meal, and falls. This occurs commonly in older people and although the pathophysiology remains unclear, some factors have been identified leading to postprandial hypotension, including impairments in sympathetic and baroreflex function (contributes to regulating the blood pressure), gastric distension (bloating of the stomach) and release of vasodilatory peptides (causes widening of the blood vessels).

Currently there is no consensus in the literature regarding the association of cardiac arrhythmias with falls. The difficulty in making this link arises from the fact that the 24-hour ambulatory echocardiogram test commonly performed to detect the presence of arrhythmias is not sensitive enough for intermittent arrhythmias. More prolonged recordings are needed to detect these occasional rhythm disturbances. A recent study found older people with atrial fibrillation were more likely to have a fall, but more studies are needed to clarify this relationship.

Congestive heart failure is where the heart's pumping power is weaker than normal and can cause swollen legs and ankles, shortness of breath, fatigue, weakness and dizziness that might lead to loss of balance and falls. The common symptom of coronary artery disease is angina and this can cause a heart attack, arrhythmias and congestive heart failure, so it is another condition that puts you at risk of falls.

Falls assessment, treatment and therapies

By now you will appreciate how maintenance of posture, balance and gait is essential to safe independent living. Loss of balance causes falls and fractures resulting in loss of activity, earning and productivity. With an active ageing population, falls pose a huge challenge to society and health care and is described as one of the six 'giants of geriatrics'. The human cost of falling to the individual includes distress, pain, injury, loss of confidence and loss of independence, as well as affecting relatives and carers.

Polypharmacy (the use of a large number of medications) is one of the major contributory factors towards falls in older people. Common culprits are antidepressants, sleeping pills, tranquillizers, antipsychotics, blood pressure tablets and anticonvulsants.

It is therefore essential that healthcare professionals are aware of the possible risks of falls in older people and actively enquire about and record the falls episodes in the previous twelve months. They should also enquire about any changes in posture, gait, balance and stability.

As part of your multifactorial falls assessment your doctor would normally assess gait, balance, mobility, muscle strength, neurology, cognition, environment, activities of daily living, functional ability and fear of falls.

If you experience falls, you may be referred to the local falls service. They may address strength and balance training, home hazard assessment and intervention, vision correction and medication review and modification. Increasingly 'gamification of therapy' with 'exergames' – video game-based balance and stability exercises – are being recommended as an enjoyable, engaging home or community-based therapeutic regime.

Awareness, advice, reduction of modifiable risks and exercise-based strength and balance training are proven to be most beneficial in falls prevention.

Exergames

Our unit in Sheffield undertook a feasibility study on the relative effectiveness of commercially available video-based balance games (the Nintendo Wii Fit in this case) when compared to traditional balance rehabilitation exercises (the Cawthorne Cooksey balance exercises). The study design was a randomized controlled trial where individuals were randomly allocated to either the Wii Fit or the exercise arms of the trial for six weeks. They also completed validated balance and general well-being questionnaires and had their visual fields mapped before and after the six weeks.

The results were very encouraging. Most of the patients in the Wii Fit group noticed an improvement in their balance and stability compared to the Cawthorne Cooksey exercise group. Their visual fields also showed a significant improvement in this period. However, these gains wore off when the patients stopped using the games after six weeks. Hence we always advise continued engagement with balance rehabilitation exercises to receive sustained benefits.

Neville

An 86-year-old man was referred to the neurotology department at the hospital, his doctor stating, 'Please see this gentleman who is complaining of persistent "dizziness" over the last year and a half.' On closer questioning he had also been experiencing sudden vertigo on changing posture and had fallen twice in the last year, resulting in a dislocated shoulder on one occasion.

Neville was hypertensive and diabetic, smoked 30 roll-ups and had a glass of whisky per day. He lived alone in a bungalow. He was on eight different medications, including those for blood pressure and diabetes, painkillers for arthritis, sedatives, aspirin, statins and laxatives.

A comprehensive multidisciplinary assessment was undertaken. This showed lower limb muscle weakness and wasting, loss of sensation in the soles of both feet and evidence of poor blood sugar control over the last six months. Balance assessment revealed poor static balance and sway and a prolonged 'time up and go' test (more than 12 seconds). Most interestingly, however, a Dix-Hallpike positional test unmasked an undiagnosed BPPV (see Chapter 8). This was immediately corrected with an Epley manoeuvre with complete resolution.

Based on the responses to the 'fear of falls' questionnaire, a detailed discussion was undertaken, backed up by an occupational therapist's assessment of his home environment, with measures introduced to remove falls hazards. A full medication review and modification was also undertaken, with a reduction in the total number of his daily medications from eight to four.

Lifestyle modifications were advised and monitored via primary care with a drastic reduction in his smoking and alcohol intake (total cessation was deemed an unrealistic and unachievable target due to these being long-established habits). He was also enrolled in group exercise sessions, initially by the hospital falls service and then in the community. Neville has remained self-caring and has not had any falls in the last two years.

6

Medicines

Polypharmacy – too many medicines?

One of the most common causes of imbalance is 'polypharmacy', but this is often disregarded or ignored. Polypharmacy is when a person takes five or more medicines. When different drugs are taken together they can work against each other and affect their ability to work as they were intended to. They can either be synergistic (one drug can make the other stronger) or antagonistic (one drug may reduce or cancel out the other). It is not exactly known what effect it has on people when they take several medicines. However, it can be very harmful for older and frail people and those with multiple medical issues.

It is now known that if you take four or more medicines daily you have an increased possibility of falls. Also, 81 per cent of people who take six or more medicines are three times more likely to have a drug reaction.

Doctors and patients should still prescribe and take medicines when they are required. Medication plays an important role in treating sudden illness and keeping long-term conditions under control. It is important that your individual circumstances and history are carefully considered. The best way to avoid drug interactions is to be on the lowest possible dose of as few medicines as possible. It is good practice to have your prescription reviewed regularly and stop medicines that are not essential.

The following medications can commonly cause drug-induced imbalance:

- antihypertensives (blood pressure)
- anticonvulsants
- antidiarrhoeals
- antivertigo medications
- anxiolytics and antidepressants

- chemotherapeutic
- diuretics
- drugs with Parkinsonian effects
- sedatives.

Postural drop in blood pressure

Medicines often cause an abnormal drop in blood pressure (ortho-static hypotension). Many individuals who experience this side effect can feel lightheaded or dizzy when they stand up from sitting or lying down. Sometimes doctors prescribe antivertigo medication for this rather than looking to see if this is being caused as a side effect of medication. Doctors should realize that new or recent balance symptoms could be related to a change in prescribed medications. This should lead them to review the medicines you are taking. Sedatives (medications with calming effects, such as benzodiazepines) and antipsychotics (barbiturates, phenothiazines, amitriptyline) can make older people confused and lead to falls and hip fractures.

Chemotherapeutics and antibiotics

Elements of drugs used for chemotherapy to treat cancer, such as cisplatin and vincristine, can harm hearing and balance. The damage can permanently affect both ears, although this is not very common.

Some antibiotics, such as aminoglycosides like gentamicin or streptomycin, can damage the balance structures inside the ear. This can cause people to lose their balance altogether. However, this depends on the dose so it is possible to stop these effects if it is caught early enough in the course of the antibiotics.

Drug withdrawal and pharmacokinetics

All medicines behave differently; they enter the circulation in vary-ing proportions and are their most effective at different levels. Doctors need to keep a close eye on this and adjust accordingly. Older people have a reduced reaction to changes in blood pressure and plasma volume (plasma is the largest component of human blood). They can also have bigger and more pronounced side effects

with changes in medication. For example, quickly stopping sedative medicines (in the benzodiazepine group) can cause confusion
and fits, and if beta blockers are suddenly stopped this can lead to
tachycardia (a racing heartbeat) and some heart conditions.

Over-the-counter medicines

Sometimes people don't tell their doctor if they are taking medicines they have bought themselves. Even common medicines, such
as painkillers, cough medicine, anti-dizziness and travel sickness
medicine or antidiarrhoeals in irritable bowel syndrome, can cause
lightheadedness. It is therefore important to tell your doctor, and
your doctor to ask you, about any over-the-counter medicines that
you may be using regularly as this could be contributing to your
balance problems.

7

Balance disorders in children and teenagers

Fortunately, balance problems are rare in children. Children also recover much faster than adults. Balance disorders are difficult to diagnose in children as they cannot describe their symptoms very well and they do not always report them. It is therefore necessary for doctors to ask very focused questions of both the child and the parent/guardian in order to understand what the symptoms are.

Common conditions that might result in balance disorders

Otitis media (glue ear)

Children with glue ear are often described as 'clumsy' by their parents. They tend to bump into things and fall over. Their symptoms can change depending on whether there is fluid trapped behind the ear drum or not (this is called middle ear effusion).

Benign paroxysmal vertigo of childhood

This is a type of migraine that can occur in childhood. It is short-lasting and symptoms include sweating, nausea, paleness and balance problems, but not necessarily headaches. Many children who have BPVC go on to experience full-blown migraine in adulthood. Migraine with dizziness is common in teenage girls.

Trauma

Trauma, especially a head trauma, can cause labyrinthine concussion or brain injury, which means that there can then be symptoms of different types of balance conditions. This is extremely important in children who have large vestibular aqueduct syndrome (LVAS) and gradual worsening of hearing and balance each time they have an attack, even after a minor head trauma, such as heading a football.

The loss of hearing is usually sensorineural (this means it affects the inner ear rather than the outer or middle ear), which can first be seen in childhood and sometimes gradually gets worse to a point where it can reach total deafness in adulthood. The balance symptoms can vary from slight imbalance to episodes of dizziness, which may last for different periods of time. Even though there may be symptoms, balance function can be normal when tested until adulthood. There is also a link with Pendred syndrome (a genetic disorder with hearing loss, enlarged thyroid and large vestibular aqueducts) and Mondini malformations (a type of inner ear malformation).

Neurodegenerative conditions

Neurodegenerative conditions such as familial ataxia or encephalopathy start with gradual balance symptoms. Central nervous system abnormalities, such as rare tumours like neurofibromatosis type 2 (NF2), can also start in the same way.

Congenital vestibular loss

Congenital vestibular loss can occur on its own or linked with maternal infections, such as congenital cytomegalovirus, or as part of other conditions, such as Usher syndrome (progressive deafness and blindness due to abnormal pigment deposits at the back of the eye). Conditions linked to chromosomal abnormalities often have developmental abnormalities connected with the vestibular system. Down's syndrome can be connected with abnormalities of the inner ear balance organs – a large vestibule and changes in the semicircular canals. Some familial conditions may include a malformed vestibule. Alport syndrome (a genetic condition where hearing loss is associated with kidney disorders) and Chiari malformations (a small area of herniation of the back of the brain into the spinal column) can also involve an abnormal or hypoplastic sac and/or vestibular aqueduct. A broad variety of deformities linked with the endolymphatic sac and ducts in the inner ear balance apparatus are associated with hereditary conditions such as Klippel-Feil (abnormal joining of two or more spinal vertebrae in the neck), Usher, Apert (abnormal early fusion of skull bones), Waardenburg (people have pigmentary abnormalities causing an isolated white forelock or differently coloured eyes), Marfan (often tall and thin with a disorder of the connective tissue affecting the joints), Paget (abnormal thickening of skull bones) and Pendred (hearing loss and goitre with hypothyroidism) syndromes.

Katie

Katie, 29, was a PhD student who experienced a sudden total loss of hearing in her right ear. Her hearing had been gradually deteriorating for 15 years, beginning when she was 14. She had been wearing a hearing aid for five years and her hearing had been slightly reduced on both sides for two years. She used to play hockey and was a black belt in judo, but had not played contact sports for ten years.

Neurotological examination did not reveal any abnormalities. A high-resolution CT scan showed large vestibular aqueducts on both sides. All other tests to look for the syndromes described previously were negative. The test results and consequences were discussed with her and she was informed that it was possible she could have further loss of hearing and she should be careful to avoid minor bumps to the head. She carried on wearing the hearing aids in one ear (although she struggled with this) and she completed her PhD.

When her hearing got worse in the left ear, she qualified for a cochlear implant, which was fitted when she was 34 years old. Now she works as a computer analyst for a multinational company and has two young children who have normal hearing and balance.

How to assess a child with balance problems

It is very important to remember that children may use a completely different vocabulary to describe their balance symptoms compared to adults. It is also important to interact with the child in an empathic manner and not be dismissive of his or her symptoms. Parents and other adults often tend to err on either end of the spectrum – that is, either being dismissive or overprotective. Neither of these is helpful as it can only confuse the picture and lead the doctor down the wrong track.

The first step is to determine if there is a 'spinning sensation' (rotatory vertigo, which is very likely to come from the inner ear) or something completely different that may be showing as dizziness. How long the symptoms last varies depending on the condition so, for example, in BPPV they can last from seconds to minutes, but in migraine or labyrinthitis it could be hours or even days.

Other symptoms can also give early signs: sweating, palpitations and rapid breathing may be due to panic attacks; hearing loss and tinnitus may be due to ear disease, such as otitis media (glue ear) or cholesteatoma; headaches or visual problems may be due to migraine. Motion sickness can also be linked to migraine, family history of autoimmune conditions or inner ear brain tumours that may affect the younger generation.

Some rarer conditions to consider in childhood dizziness are Gorlin syndrome, NF2 or LVAS.

It is also important to look out for other deep-rooted psychological issues that may make the child fake balance symptoms to get attention – medical or otherwise. This needs to be taken into account when the symptoms do not tie up and test results do not show anything. Doctors and parents/guardians should not ignore the child's complaints when there is no clear diagnosis. The child's worries should be taken seriously and help and support offered. It is crucial that emotional, physical or psychological abuse should be ruled out. If this is suspected, then safeguarding should be put in place.

Physical examination of children must be adapted depending on their age, level of understanding and how good they are at following instructions. Older children can be examined and tested in the same way as adults, but examining younger children needs to be tailored to them so that they will cooperate fully and not feel anxious.

The ears need to be examined to check for infection, inflammation or disease. One of the most important clues is the eye movements. Jerky, uncontrolled eye movements (nystagmus) can be linked to disorders that cause inflammation of the ear (such as severe otitis media or labyrinthitis) or disease in the brain. Downward beating nystagmus (when the eyes drift upwards and 'beat' or jump downwards) should arouse suspicion of there being a problem with the brain, such as compressive Chiari malformation, which is when there is a herniation of the brainstem producing pressure on the neurons. Inherited nystagmus that has been present since birth should also be taken into account. In children this tends to be random, can be in any direction and does not cause any symptoms.

The Romberg or Fukuda stepping test are used in adults to check for postural stability. Walking tests appropriate to age can be used to look for ataxia. The Dix-Hallpike positional test can be used to exclude BPPV.

Are detailed investigations always necessary?

Most of the diagnosis can be made by asking specific questions and undertaking an assessment. Elaborate tests usually cause unnecessary distress for the child and may overemphasize the possibility of an organic cause in the absence of one. Some children, however, will need full otoneurological assessment and objective balance tests, such as videonystagmography, computerized dynamic posturography and rotation chair testing. They should also have some form of scan to rule out problems with the brain. Blood tests are only done if there is a possibility the person could have certain genetic or autoimmune diseases.

What can be done for a child with a balance disorder?

The good news is that children make good recoveries from short-lasting balance problems. Children are more adaptable than adults in managing their balance symptoms. There is not very much literature about vestibular conditions in children, however, and people tend to look to the adult population to understand it. Therefore, there is little data and outcomes and knowledge vary from one hospital to another. Also, a lot of the disorders in children start differently from how they start in adults.

It is difficult to test children, particularly younger ones. Sometimes it can be very difficult to get accurate details of the problem from the child or his or her parent/carer. Children with balance disorders often describe their symptoms very differently from adults and use very different descriptors for their symptoms. It is therefore important to be in tune with a child's way of thinking. He or she can feel isolated and limited due to the symptoms. It is important to remember that severe balance problems can be very frightening to a child and the family. It is therefore essential to be understanding, empathetic and reassuring to gain their trust.

Another issue is that adolescents may report dizziness as a way to attract medical attention for some deeper underlying personal problem, such as bullying. Doctors should approach reaching a diagnosis in the same way that they would in any other case.

Ideally children with balance problems should see a specialist

ENT doctor and an audiologist with an interest in and experience of children. Sometimes many specialists and agencies dealing with a child will need to be involved. It is crucial in such situations to show compassion to children and their families in order for them to be treated successfully.

Once assessment is complete, it is important to give children and their families a clear explanation of what is happening. Balance conditions tend to resolve on their own, so it is helpful to be positive and reassure the children and parents about this.

Physical therapy has tended to be the go to treatment for lots of vestibular conditions. However, it might be that using gamification and exergames (such as the Nintendo Wii Fit balance games) is a simpler, more engaging, fun option for children than are other options. Because individuals find these enjoyable alternatives to traditional therapies, they tend to engage with them and comply better. They can also give an indication of how well people follow medical advice and what impact they have.

Individuals should given advice on measures they can take to change the possibility of developing further balance problems, such as avoiding repeated bumps to the head in LVAS and diet and lifestyle changes in migraine.

Parents and carers are keen to know how long children are likely to have these conditions as they often impact or influence future career choices. It is important that this is made as clear as possible.

8

Assessment of balance and stability

The mainstay of assessment of balance is a detailed history supported by a thorough examination. Expensive and time-consuming tests only help confirm the diagnosis but are not absolutely essential to arrive at a diagnosis. The headings that follow aim to help develop a structured approach to balance assessment. More importantly, it is also to provide a self-help strategy for those with balance issues to self-assess their conditions to some extent in a systematic way and be better informed to direct their enquiries in the right direction.

What to ask in the history of someone with a balance disorder?

Taking a detailed medical history with detective-like inquisitiveness and precision is the key. Balance symptoms are described in many different ways. For example, people may say, 'I experience dizziness, giddiness or vertigo' or they may say they have 'lightheadedness', 'a muzzy head', 'a fuzzy head', 'spinning', 'floaty sensation' or 'I feel as if I am walking on clouds.' It is essential to separate the symptoms of rotatory vertigo, as in MD or BPPV, from persistent imbalance, as in vestibular failure.

It is also crucial to establish the duration as well as the precise onset of balance symptoms. Certain disorders, such as labyrinthitis, MD or BPPV, usually start with a memorable (in the most unpleasant sense) and violent episode that the person can recall accurately. The duration of episodes of severe vertigo can vary from minutes to hours to days, whereas symptoms in conditions with progressive balance loss, as in some neurological conditions or ageing, are constant and develop slowly.

It is then necessary to establish any triggers or relieving factors. For example, certain conditions, such as MD and vestibular migraine, can be triggered by some food ingredients, while conditions such as BPPV can be triggered by a change in position or, in the case of visual vertigo, by a visually challenging environment. Certain conditions, such as labyrinthitis or VN, can be preceded by viral illnesses, and BPPV by whiplash or a head injury. Sometimes balance symptoms may be associated with ear infections or ear discharge. The symptoms recurring at intervals are also another pointer towards a diagnostic label. Conditions such as MD can occur in relapsing and remitting bouts and some attacks can come in clusters. Similarly, they may be associated with periods of hormonal fluctuation or fluid retention, such as with the menstrual cycle. Many people have a chronological diary of balance episodes. Some offer these voluntarily at the time of consultation. They provide a valuable insight into the impact the condition is having on the person's life and also show any patterns that may not be obvious.

It is very important to enquire about and record any falls as a result of balance episodes and any fragility fractures resulting from them.

Associated symptoms are also quite important. For example, MD may be associated with one or more of hearing loss, tinnitus, fullness of the ears, nausea and vomiting. However, conditions such as BPPV and VN may not be associated with any additional symptoms.

Medications and alcohol can exacerbate some of these symptoms, which can be compounded in the presence of other chronic conditions such as diabetes, hypertension, coronary heart disease, movement disorders and other neurological conditions.

Previous ear surgery or a head trauma may leave a person with chronic balance problems. Sometimes operations such as mastoidectomy (operations on the middle ear to clear infections), stapedectomy or ossiculoplasty (operations to replace the little bones of hearing in the middle ear) may result in short-term reduction in balance, which usually improves with time. Certain operations, such as labyrinthectomy and vestibular neurectomy, are specifically designed to eliminate the offending balance apparatus or nerve supply and may therefore leave the individual with a permanent loss of balance function on the operated-on side. Prior knowledge of the function in the unaffected side is very important before undertaking any procedures on the opposite ear that may inadvertently render the person disabled.

A past medical history of conditions such as migraine can predispose an individual to MD or vestibular migraine. Similarly, many individuals with MD often have a strong family history of MD or migraine (see Chapter 3). This is only a correlation and, as yet, there is no strong evidence to point towards a genetic cause or inheritance of this condition.

Examination

All patients need a thorough ENT and neurotological examination. The ears need to be examined in detail for structural anomalies that may be either from birth or acquired later due to trauma, disease or surgery. Blockage to the ear canal can produce hearing loss as can perforation of the eardrum or disruption to the ossicles (ear bones). Diseases behind the eardrum and in the middle ear with infections or erosive conditions, such as cholesteatoma, may also cause imbalance. Concomitant nasal conditions, such as polyps, can also cause middle ear problems resulting in hearing loss that may not be directly related to the imbalance.

Following this it is important to examine all the cranial nerves in detail. Of the twelve cranial nerves the third to the eighth are most important. The third, fourth and sixth cranial nerves are responsible for the eye movements that are so important in maintaining gaze stability that in turn is essential for maintaining posture and balance. Infections or diseases of the deep part of the bone housing the ear (referred to as the petrous apex) can interfere with the functioning of these nerves resulting in a squint. The fifth cranial nerve supplies the chewing muscles and also facial sensation. It can be involved late in very large inner ear tumours (vestibular schwannoma), which can cause simultaneous loss of balance. It can also be involved in painful neuralgias, such as trigeminal neuralgia, which can, in rare situations, cause diagnostic confusion with vestibular migraine. The seventh cranial nerve supplies muscles of facial expression and taste. This runs an interesting tortuous course in the inner ear and in the middle ear before leaving the skull behind the jawbone to supply each side of the face. It can be affected by inner ear tumours as well as erosive middle ear diseases, such as cholesteatoma, resulting in a weakness of the facial muscles, which can often confuse the picture, being mistaken for a stroke. The eighth cranial nerve is a double nerve that supplies the hearing (cochlear) and the balance (vestibular) organs separately. Tumours of the inner ear or lesions deep in the brainstem can affect this nerve.

The cerebellum is the other important structure at the back of the brain that can cause shooting pains in the face and cheek with triggers such as touch, pressure or change in temperature. It maintains both coordination and equilibrium, so plays a crucial role in maintenance of posture and balance. Hence it is important that this vital part is assessed carefully in people with balance disorders. It can be affected by tumours, trauma or stroke. This can result in subtle changes in movements, leading to differences in a person's handwriting or walking pattern or difficulty drinking out of a cup. These subtle signs can be easily missed if one is not thinking of them or looking for them specifically. The history once again is relevant here as questions directed to the partner or accompanying relative may bring to light some of these slowly developing changes that the person may be completely unaware of.

Another important examination is that of the eye. Different patterns of eye movements give invaluable clues to various balance disorders which are often associated with involuntary eye movements. Rhythmic involuntary eye movements are called nystagmus. Central nystagmus can be due to problems in the higher centres of the brain, have no specific pattern and will continue indefinitely without provocation. Peripheral nystagmus, in contrast, arises directly from the balance apparatus and is thought to be the body's compensatory mechanism to counteract the illusion of movement brought on by the irritation of the balance nerve. For example, individuals with BPPV have a classic rotatory nystagmus directed to the undermost ear when lying down along with a sudden onset of spinning sensation and nausea. This starts within forty seconds of change in posture and usually stops within a minute. This can be elicited by assuming the same position but repeated testing will fatigue the system with the disappearance of the sign for some time.

After this the next steps are to assess the dynamic stability when the person is up and about.

Diagnostic tests

Romberg, tandem gait and Unterberger tests

The Romberg test involves standing on one spot with the eyes closed and an estimate is made of the overall sway of the patient.

Then the walking pattern is assessed both at normal walking pace and with a 'heel to toe' tandem walk. Individuals with loss of function of both balance organs find it impossible or very difficult to perform this test.

The other very useful test is the Unterberger test, which involves marching on the spot with the eyes closed and hands outstretched in front. After marching on the spot for about a minute, individuals with unilateral losses rotate to various degrees. The direction of rotation is not diagnostic of the side or site of the pathology but gives an indication of the asymmetric nature of the balance loss.

Time up and go test

This test is used widely to assess older people and is very easy to undertake. The usual measure for those above 60 years of age is 9–10 seconds. The other tests that are useful in this category are the functional reach and the one-leg stand.

Retropulsion test

The retropulsion test is a very useful assessment for postural stability and an indirect indicator of the risk of falling especially in people with neurological and movement disorders. This involves a sudden unexpected shoulder pull from behind and an estimation of the ability of the individual to maintain upright posture. More than two steps backward to maintain posture is considered abnormal.

Dix-Hallpike test

BPPV is very common in older individuals and often the history may be overshadowed by the history of generalised imbalance. It is therefore important to undertake a Dix-Hallpike positional test in these people to unmask BPPV (see Chapter 3).

If positive, an Epley manoeuvre can be undertaken at the same time thus correcting a major contributory factor towards instability. An Epley manoeuvre can also be done at home with instruction (see Chapter 3).

Instrumented tests and balance laboratory tests

The quintessential laboratory test of vestibular function has been the caloric reflex test. This was discovered by Robert Bárány who won the Nobel Prize for Physiology/ Medicine for this (see later in the chapter). The test involves irrigation of the external ear canal (provided the ear drum is intact) with warm and cold water to elicit involuntary reflex eye movements (nystagmus). Warm water produces eye movements directed towards the same side as the ear being stimulated, while cold water produces the opposite effect. This tests what is known as the vestibulo-ocular reflex (VOR) (implying the linkage between the vestibule or the inner ear balance organ and the eyes). In the absence of an intact ear drum this test is performed with warm air only.

The subject has to lie with the head raised 30 degrees from the horizontal. This places the horizontal semicircular canal in a vertical position and is thought to optimize the movement of inner ear fluid called endolymph within the canal. The water temperatures used are 30°C and 44°C (37 ± 7°C), that is, 7° above or below normal body temperature.

Various instrumented tests are being proposed for quick, easy and objective measurement of balance and stability without the need for complex, expensive and time consuming laboratory tests. Some of these can be undertaken both in a balance laboratory and in the outpatient clinics with appropriate support.

The video head impulse test, as developed by Michael Halmagyi, is one such test that can be deployed quickly in an outpatient setting to acquire accurate and objective measure of the function of all balance apparatus including the function of the six semicircular canals individually (three semicircular canals on each side). The person sits facing forward with their gaze fixed at a reference point while the tester standing behind moves the head in the plane of each semicircular canal. An infrared camera built into the goggles, which the person wears, picks up the eye movements. These eye movements are then analysed by a computer programme to report on the integrity of each semicircular canal in a graphic form.

Radiology imaging

Appropriate scans may be needed to rule out any disease, such as erosive conditions (cholesteatoma, for example), structural anomalies (SSCD, for instance), developmental or congenital anomalies (such as LVAS or Mondini malformations of the inner ear, tumours, infarcts, aneurysms or vascular loops). It may also be necessary to look at the cervical spine and the major blood vessels in the neck for changes in their diameter due to, for example, carotid artery stenosis. An MRI scan usually provides maximum detailed information but, on occasion, an HRCT scan may be needed to look out for bony abnormalities. On rare occasions, specific protocols such as diffusion-weighted MRI imaging or contrast studies may be needed to look out for specific conditions. It is important to remember that these scans can be quite complicated and may bring out many incidental findings, such as white matter changes, cerebral atrophy or ischaemia sometimes associated with ageing. Therefore, it is important to provide the radiologist with as much clinical information as possible and also to cross-check the report with a specialist neuroradiologist.

Historic note

The role of the vestibular system in maintaining balance was demonstrated by Pierre Flourens, who in 1842 showed that damage to the posterior semicircular canals in pigeons caused them to fall over backwards. Charles Brown Sequard in 1860 demonstrated that cooling the inner ear balance organ (labyrinth) induced vertigo.

The highest honour for discovering the caloric reflex, however, went to Robert Bárány in 1914. Robert Bárány was the eldest of six children in an Austro-Hungarian Jewish family. Having practised as an otologist in Vienna after graduating in medicine from Vienna University in 1900, he had apparently requested to be an understudy to the legendary Sigmund Freud but was rejected by the latter who considered him 'too abnormal'. Like all great discoveries, he chanced on an observation that when he syringed cold water into the ear canal of individuals they experienced vertigo and showed involuntary jerky eye movements. The direction of the nystagmus reversed if he used warm water instead of cold in the same ear. He postulated that the caloric effect due to the temperature differential between the fluids in the inner ear and that in the ear canal caused the inner ear fluid to rise or sink inside the closed vestibule. This resulted in an illusion of vertigo and created the involuntary eye movements that could be recorded. The nystagmus provided the first surrogate objective measure of the inner ear balance organ that could be used to quantify the balance function.

Bárány served as a civilian doctor in the Austrian army during the First World War. He was captured by the Russians and was a prisoner of war at the time when he won the Nobel Prize, in 1914, so received it after his release in 1917.

Fitzgerald and Hallpike subsequently refined the test by describing the optimum position for caloric tests as 30 degrees above horizontal and water temperatures as 30 °C and 44 °C (37 ± 7 °C).

9

Newer tests

With people living longer and the rising cost of health and social care, research into vestibular conditions is gathering pace. With increased investment in balance research there is considerable potential of finding newer tests and treatments. Much is likely to be achieved in the years to come with continual advancements in technology.

Gadolinium enhanced MRI of the inner ear

This is an area of research into vestibular conditions that is very promising. Interestingly, we have known about MD for over a hundred years, but there was no impartial test to confirm the diagnosis. Thus the doctor still depends on the history that you give to arrive at the diagnosis. Equally, it is difficult to confirm or refute the diagnosis if the person makes up the symptoms. The closest we have come is electrocochleography (see later in this chapter), but the results still vary. Imaging the inner ear and balance organ with a contrast such as gadolinium (when injected into the body it enhances and improves the quality of MRI) is very encouraging and may be the answer to our search for a specific test for diagnosing MD. If the results are repeatedly reliable then this test could transform the diagnosis of one of the most life-changing vestibular diseases. Around 2004, tests on animals where gadolinium was injected into the middle ear space through the eardrum started taking place. Animals who had swollen inner ears (endolymphatic hydrops) had bulging of one of the partitions of the fluid components of the inner ear (Reissner's membrane). It is possible that the gadolinium went into the perilymph (inner ear fluid in a compartment outside separate from the endolymphatic space) and did not spill on to the endolymphatic compartment, and this was later confirmed on pathology specimens. This therefore means that there is a real possibility that this could be a diagnostic test for MD.

Trials on humans were described in a paper by Naganawa and Nakashima (2008) and were followed by other publications from other centres. Most of the studies were done using 1:8 dilution of gadolinium in normal saline with the solution being injected transtympanically (into the middle ear). A 3 Tesla machine (high-power MRI scanner) was used in most of the studies. However, acceptable results were also found using the more standard 1.5 Tesla machine. Ongoing research will allow precise diagnosis, classification and prognosis of endolymphatic hydrops and other conditions of the inner ear which have not yet been seen on scans.

The original method was to dilute the gadolinium eightfold and inject it into the middle ear with a very fine needle. The inner ear was then imaged by MRI 24 hours after the injection. It is now possible to image the inner ear after injecting the gadolinium in the normal fashion when looking for other neurological disorders of the ear.

Scanning for SSCD

Until the arrival of high-quality radiological imaging with 3D reconstruction, the condition of SSCD had been difficult to find. Previously, if you went to the doctor with these symptoms he or she would not be able to find the exact cause for them and could sometimes think that you were imagining them. But now it is possible to take images of the delicate balance organs in great detail and then make a 3D reconstruction to show the lack of bone between the balance apparatus and the brain. These HRCT scans (with enhanced imaging) are perfect for identifying this condition.

Nowadays, to confidently diagnose SSCD, it is necessary to see dehiscence on radiology. It is also crucial for you to experience typical symptoms to match the diagnosis, as well as undergoing an electrophysiological study (test of electrical activity). The radiological test of choice is still HRCT of the temporal bone (the skull bone that houses the inner ear hearing and balance organs), together with images that are rearranged in specific sections. It is believed that dehiscence can be seen in 3–5 per cent of people if high-resolution 0.5-mm CT scans are used.

If you suspect that your symptoms match that of SSCD you can request your doctor to arrange for these special scans to check this out.

Radiological evidence is crucial in diagnosing SSCD and as such plays a key part in managing the condition. Because complex surgery is an option for patients, it is particularly important that further research looks to improve the accuracy of identifying SSCD using HRCT. Recently we have published our research where we used HRCT to compare superior canal dimensions in 66 temporal bone specimens which were independently analysed by two experienced neuroradiologists. These specimens were then inspected by microscope to determine the dimensions of the bone on top of the superior semicircular canal.

Vestibular evoked myogenic potential

VEMP is a muscle response to a loud click or tone that can be measured from the eye muscles (ocular VEMP) or neck muscles (cervical VEMP). Thus if a loud noise is played into your ear then the neck and eye muscles will have a small imperceptible contraction in response to it. This, although not seen, can be picked up by electrodes placed above the relevant muscle. This goes through the vestibulo-collic reflex and is believed to measure the function of the part of the inner ear called the saccule. This is particularly interesting as up to now there have been various tests which examine different parts of the balance organ, but not the saccule.

It is easy to measure the cVEMP from the sternocleidomastoid muscle (the long muscle on the side of your neck) by using evoked response equipment (this is an electrical potential which is recorded from the nervous system by using a stimulus). It is an inhibitory response of the muscle that can be measured from a sustained contraction of the sternomastoid muscle in the neck when loud clicks or bursts of noise are played into the ear. It is present in neonates, infants and up to old age.

One of the most important ways of using cVEMP is to diagnose conditions of SSCD. There is an abnormally low threshold of cVEMP in SSCD when compared to normal. These abnormal waves return back to normal when the canal is sealed by surgery and so such a change is a way of measuring the success of surgery. cVEMP is also being explored to see if it could be used in MD where a shift in the tuning curve has been seen in the affected ear. The findings suggest that cVEMP could possibly be used to diagnose and stage the disease.

Head impulse testing

Head impulse testing is a rapid, bedside test that was first reported by Halmagyi and Curthoys (1988) and was followed by similar studies. Since then much research has been done into this which has made it an impartial way of identifying one-sided vestibulopathy (loss of function of the inner ear balance organ). The main focus of this research has been aiming to develop a standardized kit that would find, record and analyse the nystagmus by using scleral coils (track eye movements) or infrared video recordings.

The real benefit of this test is that it can check the functions of the semicircular canals in their individual planes. The device is portable and can be used at the bedside. All you need to do is sit with your head and neck relaxed and the tester stands behind you. The tester then places your head in the relevant plane for the specific semicircular canal. The head is then moved in a short, sharp jerk while the infrared camera picks up and analyses the involuntary eye movements.

Electrocochleography

Electrocochleography (ECochG) has been used for many years to study the inner ear. This involves picking up electrical responses of the inner ear as a reaction to sound stimulation of the ear being tested. The electrode can either be placed outside the eardrum or inside the middle ear in contact with the round window. Individuals who have active MD are likely to have characteristics of the response curve that is recorded after the stimulus.

Professor Gibson (2017) and his team in Sydney have done research into the use of ECochG as a way of diagnosing MD. They have published their research over the past 30 years. They developed a 'golf club' electrode that can be placed behind your eardrum under local anaesthetic. This gives a very sensitive measurement of your inner ear's responses to sound.

Gait/falls/maintenance of posture and balance

Much work is being done into the prevention of falls, particularly in older people, as this impacts greatly on their quality of life and healthcare resources. A lot of this work is done between geriatricians, physiotherapists and occupational therapists. Many randomized controlled trials are showing major benefits of personalized exercise programmes rather than generic exercises in preventing falls. Wearable technology such as smartwatches, step meters and other health bracelets and necklaces are quite commonplace. Look out for these in your surroundings over a week and make a note of how many you see. Wearable inertial sensors are now becoming very popular in gait assessment and falls prediction. Even your simple smartphone has inertial sensors and can be adapted to do some of these experiments.

The idea of using electro- or vibrotactile systems as a way of substituting vestibular function is particularly encouraging. An early prototype is a stimulator which produces an electrotacile stimulation to the tongue when it receives information from the balance sensor. As the brain is able to change and adapt it soon learns to use this extrasensory input to maintain posture and balance.

10

Rehabilitation

Dysfunction of the balance apparatus results in a loss of coordination of the systems that integrate the various inputs required to maintain your posture and stability in a static and dynamic situation. Most of the rehabilitation exercises are designed to restore this coordination. They involve a series of head, eye and body movements that pose various degrees of challenge to your system thus provoking your brain to reintegrate the input and output signals. The most commonly known exercise regime is that started by Cawthorne and Cooksey in the 1940s.

It is important to implement vestibular rehabilitation (VR) regimes early before balance function deteriorates further. This prevents your posture, balance and stability from deteriorating through progressive decompensation. Once there has been a period of prolonged decompensation you are likely to adapt your behaviour and this may have various consequences (see Table 4 for examples).

You would be ideally suited to benefit from a structured programme of VR if you have a persistent unilateral or bilateral vestibular loss or visual vertigo.

VR may also be of help if you have episodic attacks of vertigo by maintaining your current vestibular status and preventing background instability. If you have BPPV you will usually require

Table 4 Behavioural changes and some of their consequences

Behavioural changes	Unintended consequences
• Avoidance behaviour.	• Muscle stiffness, delayed compensation.
• Visual vertigo.	• difficulties in a visually busy scene.
• Increased effort.	• Headaches, tiredness.
• Anxiety.	• Palpitations, sweating, hyperventilation.
• Loss of confidence.	• Fear of falls, dependence.

specific particle repositioning manoeuvres that can be delivered by therapists or clinicians.

According to Herdman and Clendaniel (2014) the mechanism of action of VR involves retraining of the system through habituation resulting in reducing responses from repeated exposure to provocative stimuli.

What to expect when you go for VR

Prior to starting VR, the therapist will make a thorough assessment of your functional abilities and the degree and extent of the balance deficit. They will also have to take into account your age, general health, any other medical conditions and very importantly the list of medications. All these factors can contribute to increased frailty, thereby compounding your risk of falls and further disability.

After the assessment the therapist can then start a programme of VR that is tailored to your requirements.

Adaptation exercises

These exercises are designed to improve the coordination between vestibular signals and eye movements, the vestibulo-ocular reflex (VOR see Chapter 13). The exercise produces an error signal and the brain tries to correct this by improving the vestibular response (see Figure 3).

Exercises should be performed for 1–2 minutes each time. With time the therapist may introduce a different base of support, different speeds, move the target, use small/large target, plain/patterned background, sit to stand, marching, walking, jog on the spot.

Habituation exercises

The therapy is designed to produce repeated exposure to a provocative stimulus with a view to reducing the response (see Figure 4). Examples of exercises include head movements, bending forward, 180°/360° turns, reaching up and patterns, and involve five repetitions twice a day.

Gait retraining

Gait retraining includes walking at different speeds, turns, unpredictable turns, figure of eights, walking backwards/sideways, unpredictable stops, obstacles, head movements diagonally, distraction, busy environments, walk and throw a ball, walk and gaze stability.

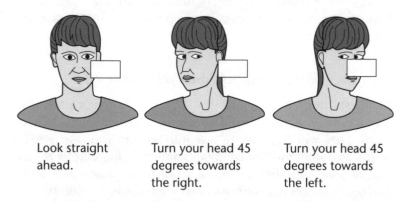

Look straight ahead.

Turn your head 45 degrees towards the right.

Turn your head 45 degrees towards the left.

Note: Business card should be positioned at eye level

- Perform for 1–2 minutes.
- Progressions: use with different base of support, different speeds, move target, use small/large target, plain/patterned background, sit to stand, marching, walking, jog on spot.

Figure 3 Adaptation exercises

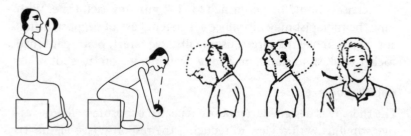

- Repeated exposure to a provocative stimulus reduces feeling of imbalance.
- Examples – head movements, bending forward, 180°/360° turns, reaching up, patterns.
- Do five repetitions three times a day.

Figure 4 Habituation exercises

Other treatments

Apart from VR, there are other exercises, therapies and treatments that can be explored. Here are some examples.

- Lower limb strengthening.
- Increase cardiovascular fitness/address deconditioning.
- Cervical spine treatment – joint mobilization, soft tissue techniques, stretches, postural advice, pain management.
- Stress management/relaxation.
- Input from a clinical psychologist.
- Visual vertigo treatment.
- Dietary changes, especially reducing coffee, additional salt, fizzy drinks and avoiding any known dietary triggers.
- Medication review with a reduction in polypharmacy.

Modern video games, some with augmented or virtual reality, can also promote adaptation and habituation in a very fun, engaging and enjoyable way. Similarly, tai chi, yoga and kinaesthetics, for example, can all help improve proprioception and core stability thus assisting with balance maintenance.

Factors that may affect your recovery

Take into account the following when assessing the effectiveness of treatments and review as required.

- **Age** While imbalance is common in older people, age itself does not reduce the chances of recovery.
- **Comorbidities** There has been very little research into comorbidities. Decreased proprioception (joint and touch sensation) with osteoarthritis, peripheral neuropathy, cataracts, diabetes, low blood pressure can restrict the ability to exercise as well as reduce balance cues.
- **Psychological factors** Anxiety, depression, poor coping strategies and lack of social support can affect outcomes. No direct association with depression and vestibular problems have been reported, but these conditions can affect recovery. Maladaptive coping strategies can also be associated with a reduced quality of life and depression.
- **Severity of deficit** Can affect recovery.
- **Medication** Vestibular suppressants can inhibit recovery.
- **Central vestibular deficits** These can also be slow to improve.

11

Neurosurgical and other treatment strategies

Dev Bhattacharyya

As you know by now, our ability to orientate ourselves, whether we are moving or standing still, relies on a complicated interaction between our visual system, proprioception and the vestibular system in the inner ear seamlessly working together and processing the information that allows us to be steady and function normally in our day-to-day life.

When you move the position of your head or turn your head, there are various pieces of information that are sent to the brain which matches this new information and makes you aware of the altered position. This allows the muscular system to make spontaneous minor adjustments to keep you steady.

Any of these systems can sustain damage for various reasons which allow a mismatch of information to be presented to your brain and the net result is that there is a mismatch between what you see and what you feel. This is often referred to as vestibule–proprioceptive mismatch. This gives rise to a sensation of dizziness or vertigo. In extreme cases this can lead to unsteady gait as well as nausea and vomiting. This can be disabling and make it difficult for you to carry out the activities of daily living or hold down a job.

As you have already found out from the previous chapters, there are many causes of dizziness ranging from diseases of the inner ear, BPPV, labyrinthitis, MD, VN and many others.

In this chapter we will focus on the types of dizziness that can be treated neurosurgically. The term neurosurgery sometimes may worry you and make you think about serious and debilitating brain tumours and brain haemorrhages. Fortunately the conditions causing balance problems are usually minor, benign (not cancerous) and not very common.

The eighth cranial nerve

Usually the abnormalities tend to be near the base of the skull which can compress or distort the eighth cranial nerve (the main nerve for hearing and balance). Our eighth cranial nerve is called the vestibulocochlear ocular nerve and is composed of the vestibular or balance nerve and the cochlear or hearing nerves. These join to form one nerve which is the eighth cranial nerve as it reaches the brainstem. The part of the skull base where this nerve runs between the brainstem and the inner ear is filled with fluid (cerebral spinal fluid or CSF) or and lies in an angle between the cerebellum and the part of the brainstem called the pons. This is therefore called the cerebellar pontine angle or CP angle for short. This nerve in its course between the brainstem and the inner ear can come into contact with some very important blood vessels that also run in the space filled with CSF. There are mainly arteries such as the vertebral artery and its branches, which supply blood to the brainstem and also to the branches that supply the eighth cranial nerve. These blood vessels supply blood to the back part of the brain.

The most common abnormalities are called acoustic neuromas and meningiomas. These are benign tumours arising from the wall of the eighth nerve itself. They are extremely slow growing and expand at a rate slower than one millimetre per year. As they grow bigger, they compress and distort the eighth nerve giving rise to dizziness and poor balance. Often this is accompanied with tinnitus and diminished hearing in that ear. Meningiomas can arise from the covering of the brain (called meninges) in this region and give rise to similar symptoms by causing pressure and distortion of the nerves.

Dizziness can also occur from disorders of the cerebellum (the movement coordinating centre at the back of your brain) and conditions affecting it, be it tumours or simple cerebellar degeneration or a blood clot. If they are present on one side, they can cause symptoms of unsteadiness and incoordination often accompanied by dizziness. Though rare, some degenerative conditions and instability in the spine in the region of the neck can also reproduce these symptoms on extremes of neck movement.

Dizziness can also occur due to benign cysts called dermoid or epidermoid cysts which are commonly found in the CP angle (as mentioned previously). This area is deep in your brain between the inner ear and the cerebellum and is traversed by the seventh (facial) and the eighth (hearing and balance) nerves. Any cyst in this area can distort and compress the eighth nerve particularly the vestibular part of the eighth nerve, leading to symptoms of extreme dizziness.

There can also be abnormalities related to blood vessels which can interfere with the blood supply of the eighth cranial nerve – arterial venous malformations or very rarely an aneurysm from one of the big blood vessels which run through the CP angle. This aneurysm can compress or distort the nerve leading to symptoms of dizziness. Thankfully, again this is very rare.

How abnormal blood vessels cause balance problems

There are several blood vessels normally running across your CP angle on each side. Sometimes these blood vessels can be enlarged or tortuous while running through this area. They then come into contact with the eighth cranial nerve resulting in compression or distortion of the nerve which can be stretched over this loop of blood vessel. The cranial nerves have an outer coating of insulation similar to an electrical wire. This insulating layer is made up of a substance called myelin. Due to the constant friction and compression of these enlarged blood vessels, and the blood flowing through it, the myelin can get compressed or even worn out exposing the actual nerve fibre to the vibrations from the blood vessel. The blood vessels commonly implicated in these balance symptoms are the posterior cerebral artery and the anterior inferior cerebellar artery.

Symptoms

Dizziness or vertigo from a surgically treatable cause usually occurs in the older age group. You may feel a sensation of vertigo or spinning, often accompanied by nausea. The symptoms fail to improve with medication used to suppress vestibular symptoms or may become worse with such treatments. The symptoms often worsen with activity or when the head or body is held in a particular position and settle with bed rest. The severe dizzy spells manifest as an unsteady gait and you may be feeling 'drunk'.

You may also notice a concomitant reduction in hearing and troublesome tinnitus.

The doctor will usually order tests to confirm the diagnosis. They include pure tone audiograms, determination of speech discrimination, brainstem auditory evoked potentials and an MRI scan.

Ben

Ben is a 51-year-old sales manager. He had left-sided pulsatile tinnitus, diminished hearing and poor balance brought on by dizziness. The symptoms started four years previously and progressed to the stage where his dizziness prevented him from driving. This affected his job and he felt his dizziness and poor balance made his gait unsteady to the extent that his colleagues enquired if he was inebriated.

An MRI scan revealed a large blood vessel impinging on the eighth nerve and distorting as it entered the brainstem.

Ben underwent microvascular decompression of the eighth nerve where the dilated blood vessel was removed from contact with the nerve. A small construct made of Teflon sponge was interposed between the nerve and blood vessel to prevent any such conflict happening again in the future.

Six weeks after surgery, the dizziness and unsteady gait had disappeared. Ben was able to drive and returned to work.

Results of surgery

The results of surgery detailed in the case study about Ben have long been established in the medical literature. In one of the earliest series, of 207 patients who underwent surgery for severe vertigo, 80 per cent were relieved of their symptoms. The risk of surgical complications is low. There is a small chance of recurrence of the symptoms some years after the operation, however. Dizziness and vertigo are relieved in a greater percentage of those affected than in tinnitus.

This kind of surgery is performed only in highly specialized centres, usually as a collaboration between an ENT surgeon and neurosurgeon specializing in this condition. Referral from the patient's own doctor to either of these specialist surgeons will set the ball rolling.

Non-surgical options

Meningiomas and acoustic neuromas respond well to stereotactic radiosurgery and a one-off treatment with the gamma knife will control the growth of these benign tumours in more than 90 per cent of patients (see Table 5).

The gamma knife works by focusing an intense beam of gamma rays (radiation) very precisely on the tumour. It is highly accurate to the order of 0.1 to 0.2 mm. The radiation damages the growing parts of the tumour and also eradicates its blood supply to stop it growing. The radiation targets only the tumour and spares the surrounding normal brain.

Table 5 Common neurological causes of dizziness and their treatment

Neurological cause of dizziness	Preferred treatment	Doctor
• Meningioma, acoustic neuroma.	• Stereotactic radiosurgery with gamma knife or surgery.	• Neurosurgeon.
• Cysts – dermoid, epidermoid.	• Surgery.	• Neurosurgeon.
• Arteriovenous malformations.	• Stereotactic radiosurgery with gamma knife or surgery.	• Neurosurgeon.
• Cerebral aneurysm.	• Coiling or surgery.	• Neuroradiologist or neurosurgeon.
• Compression of nerve by blood vessel.	• Surgical decompression of the nerve.	• ENT surgeon or neurosurgeon.

12

Psychological factors

Dr Jo Sessions

There has been a crossover between medical and psychological explanations for our experience of balance difficulties as far back as the 1800s. There were fewer such multifactorial explanations during the period of rapid scientific discoveries and medical specialization in the early 1900s. More recently, attention has started to focus again on this area and what is apparent is that psychological factors play a significant role in dizziness for many people. In this chapter we will look more closely at the relationship between balance difficulties and the impact of these psychological factors.

As you already know, symptoms of dizziness are far more common than is widely assumed and thought to affect around 30 per cent of the population. Within this group there is significant variation in the forms these balance difficulties can take, from MD, visual vertigo, vestibular migraine, labyrinthitis and BPPV to symptoms of dizziness that do not have an established medical diagnosis but are recognized by practitioners as chronic subjective dizziness or phobic postural vertigo.

This heterogeneity leads to considerable variation in the way we perceive our dizzy symptoms and how it affects us. Many of us find symptoms of dizziness an unpleasant, even scary experience and at times this can be very overwhelming.

It is not unusual for you to feel frustrated, isolated and alone if you have frequent such experiences due to balance problems. As there are no overt physical symptoms or signs apparent in those with balance disorders, the rest of the world often does not appreciate the difficulties faced by them. For instance, overly stimulating environments can often lead to persistent feelings of sickness and vomiting and you may feel fatigued due to the energy expended in overcoming the symptoms. Also, as symptoms are unpredictable, you may be worrying how others will react if you appear to be 'walking drunk' or fall or collapse while in public. You may experience constant feelings of heightened anxiety and a negative impact on your mood.

If there is no clear organic explanation for one's balance difficulty it can be perceived as malingering, which can often lead to feelings of shame. In addition, as there is very little awareness of balance conditions among friends, family and employers, it is difficult to get them to fully understand the effect of the symptoms.

It is completely understandable that people with balance difficulties will have these feelings. Many of these experiences are shared by other people with long-term debilitating health conditions.

An unfortunate consequence of these reactions to balance problems is that any such feelings and responses which increase the focus on avoiding having these experiences have a further negative impact on the balance difficulty. This sets up a negative vicious cycle.

A helpful psychological model in understanding the negative impact of feelings of anxiety and so on on the balance system and strategies to help negate these is the basis of the model of compassion focused therapy.

Bio-psycho-social model

For the purposes of this chapter we will draw on a simplified model of compassion focused therapy, originally developed by Professor Paul Gilbert (2010). One aspect of this model is its approach to understanding behaviour in terms of the influence of the limbic system. This is the emotion centre of your brain and thought to be a primitive counterpart of the more advanced, thinking centre of your brain (or cerebral cortex). The limbic system is made up of two important areas called the hippocampus and amygdala. The main function of these parts of the brain are to increase our survival by remembering events that caused strong emotions previously, and then instantly and automatically triggering a response aimed to protect us.

Research on the neurophysiology of emotion has identified three distinct emotion regulation systems, which the limbic system appears to respond differently to. These include:

- threat and protection systems, which respond through anger, anxiety and disgust;

- drive, resource-seeking and excitement systems;
- contentment, soothing and safeness systems.

The understanding behind this model is that if something in our environment is perceived as threatening – either physically, socially or psychologically – the amygdala or brain's alarm response will respond instantly and automatically create a protective mechanism to limit this threat. A defensive response is typically 'fight, flight, freeze or submit' and involves responses at the level of emotions, thoughts, behaviours and physiology.

At a physiological level a defensive response involves the stress hormone cortisol. Cortisol released into the bloodstream increases your speed of sensory response and puts the body into a state of high alert so that you are ready to respond instantly to a situation that may be perceived as a threat.

Pathways in the brain that are used more frequently start to become stronger and so more easily available. If we are faced with life situations where we are more frequently encountering threatening experiences, we tend to become vigilant to these, so that we are more likely to appraise an event as threatening and respond more quickly to it. In addition, if we have experienced unpleasant events earlier in life our threat system will remember the strong emotions attached to these events and trigger instant and automatic responses to protect against these in the future.

To respond effectively to our environment we need equilibrium in the pathways between the three affect regulation systems, which echo the neurophysiological ones:

- drive, excite, vitality
- content, safe, connect
- anger, anxiety, disgust.

The relevance of this bio-psycho-social model to understanding balance difficulties is twofold. First, it provides a broad understanding of how the multiple unpleasant experiences related to balance disorders aggravate the condition. Second, it helps us identify coping strategies to 'balance-out' the threat focus of the affect regulation systems. Balancing out the pathways in the affect system helps to increase your ability to manage unpleasant experiences and in turn address the difficulties caused by balance disorders.

How balance difficulties can be maintained

The compassion focused therapy model helps to understand how our affect system is designed to prioritize emotionally threatening experiences in order to increase our survival chances. The system then becomes faster in detecting and responding to these potentially threatening events should they recur. The implication of this, for someone with a balance disorder, is that an unhelpful cycle can be activated which, unfortunately, aggravates and perpetuates the balance problem.

It is completely understandable how a condition that limits your functioning will lead to actual feelings of sickness, disorientation and fatigue. These are again things that we will appraise negatively from a psychological and social perspective. Such negative thoughts will increase our focus on these events as threatening.

Equally, due to the central role of balance in maintaining our safety, it is also inevitable that there will be an automatic physiological threat response to any feeling of being off balance – this is an increase in autonomic arousal which increases vigilance to autonomic responses, such as balance. Unfortunately, due to the sensitizing impact of increased autonomic arousal on the balance system, this physiological response directly aggravates the balance difficulty. As a result a vicious cycle is set up whereby an already compromised balance system has an increased negative reaction to any increase in autonomic arousal. This can be triggered:

- **physiologically** an overstimulating environment, either through visual stimulus or physical stimulus with obstacles;
- **socially** 'What will others think if I wobble, fall over or collapse?';
- **psychologically** 'What use am I if I can't even get this shopping finished?'

As a result the association between balance difficulty and threat becomes increasingly powerful and established. There will be subjective variations within this threat focus depending on your previous experience of threat, the particular implications of the balance disorder for you and the existing triggers that may exist in your life already.

The implications of the compassion focused therapy model are to understand that how the majority of us respond to a balance difficulty will actually aggravate the condition and that there will be subjective variation in how balance difficulties affect different people depending on variation within their threat focus. To counteract this threat focus, the model suggests actively balancing out activities that also stimulate the drive and self-soothe affect regulation systems.

Psychological factors that can help balance difficulties

According to the compassion focused therapy model there are three main areas of the affect regulation system. We have discussed the threat-focused affect regulation system and its primitive function of increasing our chances of survival. The drive affect regulation system can be thought of as the system that motivates and directs us to important resources or life goals. The feelings associated with this system are linked to arousal, pleasure and feeling energized (in evolutionary psychology theory these are thought to develop from the emotions and motivational systems that direct animals towards important rewards and resources, such as food, alliances, procreation opportunities and nest sites). The limit the balance symptoms place on our functioning reduces the opportunity to activate this emotion regulation system in the presence of balance disorders, so we may need to stop a form of exercise or activity we enjoy or be unable to continue in the same line of work, for example.

The compassion focused therapy model suggests it would be important to consider opportunities to activate this emotion regulation system. If one has had to make changes in this area as a result of the balance difficulty, it would be useful to consider alternative goal-directed activity. Or if this is an area that has become neglected, because of the increased focus on threat and preservation, it would be useful to re-engage with it.

Alternatively, it is also possible that this focus on goal-directed behaviour that motivates us can lead to a focus on activity that is beyond realistic limits. This can then lead to fatigue, frustration and possibly a sense of failing, which has the negative consequence of fuelling the threat focus. Hence it is crucial to set realistic goals and time frames.

Self-soothing

The final emotion regulation system to be considered is the affili-
ation or self-soothing system. This is concerned with feelings of
well-being, peacefulness and contentment (non-seeking). These are
not related just to the absence of threat but appear to be qualita-
tively different from the positive feelings of the drive system. This
is our affect area which is often least attended to in a debilitating
and/or long-term health condition. For someone with a balance
difficulty, actively stimulating this area of the emotion regulation
system can be particularly helpful in balancing the increased threat
focus from the balance disorders.

Mindfulness

One strategy that can be a helpful starting point is mindfulness.
This is a technique which is being used increasingly as a self-help
strategy in many health conditions. The rationale is that mindfulness helps us to focus our minds in the here and now. Generally
speaking the things that we are most threatened by exist in the
past or the future. By actively placing the focus of your attention in
the here and now you will be providing more opportunity to access
feelings of safety and contentment. Another benefit of mindfulness
is that it increases your awareness of yourself including how you
may be feeling physically or emotionally at any given time. As a
result you are then more able to act to increase feelings of safety,
contentment or connection.

An important principle of the compassion focused therapy model
is that an imagined scenario has the same impact on brain function as does an actual scenario. For example, if you were to imagine
eating something you like, you can experience your mouth watering
in the same way that you would if the actual food were in front of
you. The rationale of the compassion focused model is that you can
stimulate an affect system by imagining a scenario that engages it.

So if you can imagine a context in which you have previously felt
soothed, content, safe or connected to others, this will stimulate the
self-soothing affect area. Another strategy that can be used as a way of
coping, to smooth out unpleasant experiences in balance difficulty, is
to actively focus your mind on a previous occasion when you have felt
content and build this into as evocative a scenario as you can.

13

Visual vertigo

Christopher Bowse

Visual vertigo was defined by Professor Adolfo Bronstein in 1995 as being a 'syndrome where symptoms are triggered or exacerbated in situations involving rich visual conflict or intense visual stimulation.'

This is sometimes loosely referred to as 'supermarket vertigo' due to the gross overstimulation of visual fields from the shelving patterns and movement of people giving rise to balance symptoms. The next time you are at a supermarket try and observe how densely packed the items on the shelves are and how complex the pattern of movement of people in the aisles are. Now imagine how it might feel if you were to have a background balance weakness but were expected to navigate your way through this crowd safely.

What causes visual vertigo?

The basic reasoning is that there is a mismatch between what the eyes are seeing and what the body is feeling. This mismatch often tricks your brain into believing that there is movement while you are actually still. Similarly, normal movement might produce an exaggerated response in an attempt to maintain balance and stability.

The symptoms may develop a few days or weeks following an acute peripheral vestibular disorder. This would be experienced as a spinning dizziness also known as rotatory vertigo. Visual problems may also cause visual vertigo or reduced sensory information from the body's skin, ligaments, muscles, tendons or joints. You are more likely to develop visual vertigo if you have a pre-existing weakness of the balance organs and rely heavily on visual clues to maintain posture and balance.

There are two main reasons visual vertigo and motion sensitivity occur.

- Motion sensitivity and visual vertigo are due to a sensory conflict or mismatch between your visual, vestibular and somatosensory systems (joints). It is thought that there is a possible discrepancy between what you expect and the actual external information that you receive.
- The combination of a vestibular disorder and subsequent visual dependence is what causes visual vertigo.

Many balance conditions can give rise to visual vertigo/motion sensitivity symptoms:

- BPPV
- labyrinthitis
- VN
- migraine-related vertigo
- MD
- head injury
- post-concussive and cervicogenic dizziness (dizziness that is worse during head movements)/whiplash-associated dizziness.

What symptoms am I likely to experience?

If you have visual vertigo you might feel tiredness, nausea, imbalance, vertigo and disorientation. Psychological disorders such as stress, anxiety, hyperventilation and panic attacks may exacerbate visual vertigo.

Your symptoms might be provoked by moving traffic, travelling in a car, boat, plane, lift or escalator, or motion of the visual surroundings, such as crowds in shopping malls.

Examples of movement in your surroundings or moving visual objects include scrolling on a PC or tablet, running water, crowds, traffic, clouds, trees, leaves or trees blowing in the wind, watching television or a motion picture. Patterns, such as stripy shirts or wallpaper, railings or the light flickering through the trees can also cause symptoms.

How is visual vertigo diagnosed?

A detailed history with the classic symptoms is the most important factor for the specialist to diagnose visual vertigo. To confirm a diagnosis, the specialist may sometimes ask you to complete some questionnaires which assess space and motion discomfort, particularly experienced in this condition.

The situational characteristics questionnaire, dizziness handicap inventory and the motion sensitivity quotient are the most frequently used tools in the diagnosis of motion sensitivity. An examination of your eye movements and other vestibular function tests can be performed to rule out central or peripheral vestibular pathology. The clinical test for sensory interaction and balance is a very important assessment tool to assess the sensory information which is received from your balance organs, visual system and information from your body which keeps your balance.

Why has my dizziness not improved?

This is due to the fact that we often naturally start to avoid certain movements which provoke further balance symptoms and make us feel worse. Often people who have dizziness or a balance problem feel frustrated as well as apprehensive. Avoidance behaviour leads to maladaptive behaviour, which is used to prevent further vertigo symptoms.

Why do some things make me feel dizzier or ill?

It is a natural tendency to avoid movements or actions that produce or exacerbate the feeling of dizziness. This is mainly because we feel that we are not in control of our surroundings. However, this only perpetuates the problem and leads to further decompensation. Recovery cannot occur if movements are avoided. The brain cannot recalibrate, learn or compensate for the changed information from your eyes, balance organs or the body. If the brain is not exposed to the sensation of dizziness, then it does not realize something is wrong and cannot begin compensation – that is, it cannot learn to recalibrate to the new information.

How is visual vertigo treated?

Treatment for visual vertigo involves customized vestibular rehabilitation as well as educating the person about compensation strategies. The three strategies used are adaptation, compensation and habituation.

Adaptation

The balance organs in both your ears normally work together as a pair. If one side stops working effectively, then there is an imbalance of information, giving rise to a feeling of rotatory vertigo so, for example, after a vertigo attack, the person might veer off to one side when walking. The brain needs to adapt to new information and adjust the balance system to these changes. Customized exercises are used to provide the brain with the information it needs to make these changes.

Compensation

There is a memory bank in your brain which stores information from your eyes, body and balance organs. If there has been an upset within the balance system, the memory bank loses information. Balance retraining exercises help to restore this information with new information which strengthens the balance system, thus reducing your sensation of vertigo and improving your balance.

Habituation

Continually repeating the actions that bring on the symptoms of dizziness or vertigo will eventually accustom the body to those actions and strengthen neural pathways.

Exercises are selected by identifying the motions and positions that provoke symptoms. Over time, with repeated motions, your vertigo symptoms will reduce so that the therapist can introduce further exercises.

It has been shown that optokinetic stimulation may be very beneficial to those who experience motion sensitivity. Repeated exposure to a DVD containing video clips of moving black and white stripes and a rotating disk for use on your PC, laptop or DVD player usually desensitizes you to the hyperstimulation that some visual environments may cause. Virtual reality (VR) and augmented reality are also proving very promising in helping to reduce visual-vestibular conflict. We have used both the Nintendo Wii Fit balance games as well as the Oculus Rift VR goggles with excellent results.

Initially you might feel a worsening of your symptoms of vertigo as the therapy kicks in. But as compensation occurs, you will progressively move from a visual dependent postural control to a more natural proprioceptive postural control with use of vestibule-proprioceptive cues.

Julie

Julie, a 24-year-old shop assistant, was diagnosed with labyrinthitis caused by an infection in her inner ear. Her symptoms were vertigo, disorientation while in the supermarket and nausea caused by eye movements such as crossing the road, watching TV or reading. She was unable to work or go out socially due to the symptoms and increasing stress levels. The initial assessment confirmed visual vertigo symptoms. She was provided with a clear explanation of the diagnosis and the cause for her symptoms. She then underwent a six week course of desensitization using traditional balance exercises, optokinetic DVDs and VR goggles. While she initially felt a worsening of her symptoms there was progressive improvement and recovery over the coming weeks. The symptoms were completely resolved by three months and she was back to her usual daily activities.

Mal de débarquement syndrome

'Mal de débarquement' is a French term that means 'sickness after disembarkation'. It has complex, undesirable symptoms, so it is termed a syndrome.

Symptoms and triggers of Mal de débarquement syndrome

Mal de débarquement syndrome (MdDS) or disembarkment syndrome is a rare neurological condition that can occur after a boat trip, aircraft flight or when the body sustains a prolonged period of movement in multiple planes of motion, simultaneously. There are also many cases when MdDS has occurred spontaneously.

Imagine stepping off a boat, plane or train and then feeling that you are constantly rocking, bobbing or swaying, like a buoy on the water in a force 8 gale. While many people experience these disorienting sensations for a few minutes after disembarking, imagine if these sensations never resolved. This is the case for people with persistent MdDS.

Although motion triggers are commonly reported, some individuals develop MdDS symptoms for other reasons including after playing computer games or having operations. An interesting feature of this condition is that individuals often feel total or partial relief from the motion sensations when they are re-exposed to passive motion, for example, when in a car or on a train. The downside to this is that when the motion stops, the severity of symptoms often increases.

It is perfectly normal for you to feel a floating, rocking or swaying sensation when getting off a boat or plane. These symptoms would ordinarily last a few hours or a few days. Sea sickness or motion sickness are obviously triggered by motion and commonly experienced. The same can occur when we are back on land, 'land sickness' or 'regaining your land legs'. It is when symptoms do not subside and potentially last for many days, months or even years that MdDS can be the cause. The presentation of MdDS symptoms tends to fluctuate and alternate from day to day. A swaying sensation may change to a rocking or bobbing sensation for no understandable reason.

MdDS is associated with a number of other symptoms, such as insomnia, headache, brain fog, blurred vision and disorientation, just to name a few. The condition can be debilitating, disabling, life-changing and may affect all aspects of people's lives.

With all balance conditions there is a physical and emotional stress which can cause anxiety. We all have life stresses to varying degrees and, when added to symptoms of MdDS, this can lead to hypervigilance and triggering of the autonomic nervous system – the fight, flight and fright response to danger. With MdDS all your balance function tests are likely to be normal. This confuses the clinician and can lead to it being labelled as a psychosomatic problem. Still today there are many who are sceptical about the diagnosis of MdDS, while many suggest that the treatments for this condition act as a placebo.

As with most rare conditions, MdDS is a complex, multi-system and multi-symptom condition and a wide range of physical/environmental factors have an impact on symptom levels. Enclosed and wide open spaces and lux level changes (lighting and illuminance) are associated with an increase in symptom severity. Hormone fluctuations, audio frequencies, 'bland' or 'busy' visual environments and changes in air pressure can also influence symptom levels. The constant feeling of being about to fall over can wreak havoc with your sympathetic and parasympathetic systems and disrupted sleep is a common feature of this syndrome. Since loss of sleep can increase symptom severity, one might sometimes feel caught in a vicious circle.

It is important for clinicians to be aware of the condition and to dispel the myth that MdDS only affects women and only occurs after disembarkation from prolonged cruises.

In some cases the onset can be what could be described as a perfect storm of events that may be a trigger for MdDS, such as two or a multitude of the following: prolonged motion, hormonal changes, anxiety, depression, triggering of the limbic system (fight, flight or fight response). Some 90 per cent of those with MdDS are women, but at present there is little evidence to support the theory that there is a hormonal link. Periods of remission can occur spontaneously or a recurrence may be triggered by events such as motion, stress or illness. MdDS can then be retriggered days, months or even years later by motion, stress or illness.

Diagnosing MdDS

Diagnosis of MdDS is usually made from the classic history and by excluding other conditions. Detailed balance testing is seldom required and can be unpleasant in this situation anyway.

Treatment options for MdDS

MdDS has been recognized and researched for decades, the cause has been elusive and researchers continue to hypothesize. Studies have suggested a link to a variant of migraine or related to motion sickness with the majority agreeing 'MdDS is a neurological condition'.

Treatment for MdDS is limited. Conventional vestibular rehabilitation can restore a sense of physical confidence but can also substantially raise symptom levels, especially if you overdo the exercises. There is good anecdotal evidence that neuro-physiotherapy is beneficial but accessing this therapy can be problematic.

Recently we have seen the development of two potential protocols for the treatment of MdDS: optokinetic stimulation and cranial stimulation.

Dr Dai's optokinetic protocol

In a study published in 1962, researchers placed volunteers in a room that rotated slowly then asked them to move their heads from side to side. The study volunteers developed unusual patterns of eye movements.

Mingjia Dai, assistant professor of neurology in New York, was interested in this paper, particularly in the types of eye movements that are a hallmark of MdDS. Dr Dai and his colleagues (2014) devised a study that supported the results of the space flight experiments and pointed to a disturbance of the VOR as the cause of the eye movements.

The VOR is a natural process by which your eyes compensate for head movements, keeping the image from becoming blurry while maintaining clear vision and spatial orientation. The VOR is an integral part of the balance system and works from a reflex from your eye (the fovea) to the inner ear balance organs.

Dr Dai hypothesized that MdDS was caused by a maladaptation of the VOR. When you are at sea, the VOR adapts to the changing, unpredictable motion in a multitude of directions. The balance system has to change its strategy to improve your stability and spatial orientation. When returning to land, the VOR does not readapt to being on land. If this hypothesis is correct, then it would seem possible to readapt the VOR. This concept led to the development of a treatment plan whereby an opposing set of visual cues and patterns of motion is used to redirect or correct the balance strategy and realign your VOR.

Initial trials involving 24 participants (21 women, three men, mean age 43.3 years) showed complete recovery or substantial improvement in 17 participants one year after treatment. Six responded well initially but their symptoms returned, and one participant received no benefit. Side effects of the treatment were negligible.

With the continued research we hope to answer a number of questions. These will hopefully include fully understanding why symptoms are relieved by motion, which neural networks are responsible for the sensation of motion and why more women than men are affected by MdDS.

Cranial stimulation

Cranial stimulation is undertaken using repetitive transcranial magnetic stimulation. In this treatment an electromagnetic field is held close to the head. This temporarily depolarizes some of the neural circuits involved and modifies the symptoms by a process called neuromodulation.

14

The future and research

Hopefully this book has given you a better understanding of balance disorders. You might also be thinking, however, is anything being done to improve your chances of recovery and offer a cure from these dreadfully debilitating conditions. There is no need to despair as lately there has been a huge amount of growth in hearing and balance research, both in Europe and the USA. We summarize here the work that is ongoing at the time of writing (see Chapter 9 for a more detailed description).

Others studies on MD

A double-blind randomized controlled trial was recently concluded by a group at Imperial College, London. This compared the effectiveness of giving gentamicin across/through the tympanic cavity versus giving steroids (methylprednisolone) via the same route. The results published in the medical journal *The Lancet* demonstrated that the steroid injection provided adequate benefit without the added risks of gentamicin. Another group in Granada, Spain are studying the genetics of MD in a large population study.

Drug trials in MD

A multicentre commerical drug trial in the USA and Europe involving injection of a medicated gel into the middle ear under local anaesthetic has produced very encouraging initial results. Further studies are ongoing in a much larger population.

Special MRI scans to diagnose MD

This test has the potential to be one of the main confirmatory tests for MD in the future. As you already know, this condition is diagnosed mainly from the symptoms and this causes a lot of

confusion and sometimes delays treatment, resulting in unnecessary suffering. Gadolinium is a dye regularly used in MRI scans.
When injected intravenously, it goes into the perilymphatic space
without spilling out on to the endolymphatic compartment,
demonstrating a bulging of the Reissner's membrane inside the
inner ear in patients with MD who have endolymphatic hydrops.

A Belgian group had initially demonstrated these results very
convincingly using more powerful 3 Tesla MRI machines. Now
equally reliable results are being seen when the 1.5 Tesla machine
is used. Wider use will allow more accurate diagnosis, classification
and prognosis of endolymphatic hydrops, as well as other conditions of the inner ear balance organs.

Functional MRI scanning in balance disorders

This test is being used more and more to look at the inner ear, most
commonly to look for areas which cause tinnitus. It is believed that
the use of this test in studying balance disorders could advance
understanding of the contribution of central pathways in balance
conditions.

Vestibular implants

These implants are based on the design of the cochlear implant. The
device which houses inertial sensor technology with gyroscopes
and accelerometers has three short electrodes which activate the
relevant vestibular nerves by stimulating the semicircular canals in
the appropriate plane of movement. It should override the abnormal
(or absent) inner ear nerve impulses to control balance symptoms
rather like an on-demand pacemaker. Following approval from the
Food and Drug Administration, some research participants have had
the implants fitted by specialists at the University of Washington
and Johns Hopkins Hospital.

Head impulse testing

As described in Chapter 9, head impulse testing can test all the
six balance canals objectively (three on each side) and is the new
way of further localizing the exact site of the deficit within the

individual balance organs. Initially researched by Halmagyi and Curthoys (1988), this is being studied and developed further to increase its application and reliability. Since then much research has been done which has made it an impartial way of identifying isolated loss of balance function in parts of the balance apparatus. Among the various techniques tested, special contact lenses with scleral coils, infrared video goggles and simple high-speed cameras are worthy of a mention.

Electrocochleography

There have been many descriptions of recording ECochG for diagnosing MD. The transtympanic 'golf club' electrode developed by Professor Gibson (2017) and his team in Sydney is inserted through the eardrum under local anaesthetic. This gives a very accurate measure of inner ear function; further refinements are ongoing.

Blood test for BPPV

Researchers in the University of Connecticut have developed a test to detect a protein (named Otolin-1) in the blood of patients with BPPV. They say that the test can be used to diagnose this common condition very early on and to keep a check on the condition. Therefore, one day in the not too distant future, you might be able to get a quick diagnosis with a simple blood test kit and then rapidly cure the balance problem yourself by doing a specific manoeuvre using a self-help video – ultimate 'patient power'.

Useful addresses

Action on Hearing loss
1–3 Highbury Station Road
London N1 1SE
Tel.: 0808 808 0123; 0808 808 9000 (textphone); 0780 0000 360 (SMS)
Email: information@hearingloss.org.uk
Website: www.actiononhearingloss.org.uk
You can download their useful factsheet on dizziness and balance problems from the website (www.actiononhearingloss.org.uk/how-we-help/information-and-resources/publications/hearing-health/dizziness-and-balance-problems).

Ménière's Society
The Rookery
Surrey Hills Business Park
Wotton
Surrey RH5 6QT
Tel.: 01306 876883
Email: info@menieres.org.uk
Website: www.menieres.org.uk/information-and-support

Vestibular Disorders Organization (VeDA)
5018 NE 15th Avenue
Portland
Oregon OR 97211
Email: info@vestibular.org
Website: https://vestibular.org

Some websites you might find useful
International Headache Society: www.ihs-headache.org/ichd-guidelines
NICE: see its Clinical Knowledge Summary for Ménière's Disease: https://cks.nice.org.uk/menieres-disease#!topicsummary
National Institute on Deafness and Other Communication Disorders (NIDCD): Glossary of common ear nose and throat terms www.nidcd.nih.gov/glossary
US National Library of Medicine: https://medlineplus.gov/dizzinessandvertigo.html

References and further reading

American Academy of Otolaryngology (1995) 'Committee on Hearing and Equilibrium Guidelines for the diagnosis and evaluation of therapy in Ménière's disease', *Journal of Otolaryngology – Head and Neck Surgery*, 113(3):181–5.

Bárány, R. (1916) 'Nobel Lecture: Some new methods for functional testing of the vestibular apparatus and the cerebellum'. Available at: <www.nobelprize.org/nobel_prizes/medicine/laureates/1914/barany-lecture.html> [accessed July 2018].

Cawthorne, T. (1946) 'Vestibular injuries', *Journal of the Royal Society of Medicine*, 39(5):270–3.

Dai, M., Cohen, B., Smouha, E. and Cho, C. (2014) 'Readaptation of the vestibulo-ocular reflex relieves the Mal de debarquement syndrome', *Frontiers in Neurology*, 5:124.

Gibson, W. P. (2017) 'The clinical uses of electrocochleography', *Frontiers in Neuroscience*, 11:274.

Gilbert, P. (2010) *Compassion Focused Therapy*. East Sussex: Routledge.

Hallpike, C. S. and Cairns, H. (1938) 'Observations on the pathology of Ménière's syndrome', *Proceedings of the Royal Society of Medicine*, 31(11):1317–36.

Halmagyi, G. M. and Curthoys, I. S. (1988) 'A clinical sign of canal paresis', *Archives of Neurology*, 45(7):737–9.

Herdman, S. and Clendaniel, R. A. (2014) *Vestibular Rehabilitation* (4th edn). Philadelphia, PA: F.A. Davis Company Publishers.

McKenna, L., Baguley, D. and McFerran, D. (2010) *Living with Tinnitus and Hyperacusis*. London: Sheldon Press.

Naganawa, S. and Nakashima, T. (2008) 'In reference to 3 Tesla delayed contrast magnetic resonance imaging evaluation of Ménière's disease', *Laryngoscope*, 118(10):1904–5.

Index

acoustic neuromas 81
adaptation exercises 77–8, 94
ageing: brain functioning and 45–8; cardiovascular system and 50–1; exergames 52; falling and 3–4, 6–7, 51–2; feedback system and 41–6; musculoskeletal system and 48–50; rehabilitation and 79
Alport syndrome 58
angiomas 83–4
anxiety xi; fear of falling 40; hyperventilation 38; stress and dizziness 5–6; visual vertigo and 92
Arnold-Chiari malformations *see* Chiari malformations
arthritis 3, 49
ataxia 39, 58
audiograms 82
autoimmune inner ear disease (AIED) 37
autophony 30

balance disorders: ageing and 40–2; assessing symptom history 63–6; bio-psycho-social model 85–7; examinations and tests 65–70; feedback system 41–6; incidence of disorders xi; neurosurgical treatments 80–3; normal balance 1–3; rehabilitation 76–9, 93–4; research and trials 100–2; symptoms of 9; testing for 71–5; vicious cycle of 88–9; *see also* dizziness; falling; medications; vertigo; *individual disorders*
Bárány, Robert 10, 68, 69–70
benign paroxysmal positional vertigo (BPPV) 10–11, 53; assessment of 63–4; blood test for 102; in children and teens 57; Dix-Hallpike test and

67–8; in older people 42; rotary nystagmus 66; visual vertigo 92
bilateral vestibulopathy 35
blood pressure 54, 64; postural drop 55; syncope 50
brain and nervous system 1, 3, 46–8, 66; ataxia 39; atypical Parkinson's disease 38–9; compression of nerves 84; cranial nerves 65–6, 81–2; examining 65–6; gait and falling 46–8; processing for balance 41; recalibrating 93; spinocerebellar ataxia 39; threat reaction 87; vertebrobasilar infarcts 22
breathing: hyperventilation 6, 38; panic attacks 59
Bronstein, Adolfo 91

Cairns, H. 13
caloric reflex test 68, 69–70
canalolithiasis 10, 11
CANVAS syndrome 36
cataracts 44
Cawthorne, T. 76
cervical spondylosis 49
cervical vestibular evoked myogenic potential (cVEMP) 31
cervicogenic vertigo 33–4
chest tightness 6
Chiari malformations 58, 60
children and teenagers: assessment and diagnosis 59–61; conditions resulting in balance disorders 57–9; treatment 61–2
cholesteatoma 60, 65, 69
Clendaniel, R. A. 77
clumsiness 22
cognitive behaviour therapy (CBT) 7
compassion focused therapy 86, 88–90
compensation 94
confusion 22
congenital anomalies 69
Cooksey, F. S. 76
cortisol 87

cranial nerve treatments 81–3
cranial stimulation 97, 98–9
cupulolithiasis 10–11
Curthoys, I. S. 74, 102

Dai, Mingjia 98
dementia 46
diabetes 6–7, 79
diet and nutrition: dizziness and 7; for Ménière's disease 15; migraine triggers 26; rehabilitation and 79
Dix-Hallpike positional test 11, 53, 60, 67–8
dizziness: bio-psycho-social model 85–7; blood vessels and 82; with BPPV 42; dealing with 7–8; experience of 5; falling 6–7; impact of 5; nervous system and 81–3; in public 85; vestibular migraine 24–6; *see also* vertigo
Down's syndrome 58

ear, inner/vestibular system 1, 2–3; ageing and 41–3; anatomy and physiology of 2–3; autoimmune disease 37; children and teens and 57–8; congenital loss 58; disorders of 10–19, 24–33; examination of 65; feedback for balance 41, 42–3; fullness in 30–1, 64; historic discoveries of 69–70; perilymphatic fistula 37–8; sensory conflicts 91–2
electrocochleography (ECochG) 71, 74, 102
encephalopathy 58
endolymphatic hydrops 13, 43, 71
endolymphatic sac surgery 18
episodic ataxia 39
Epley manoeuvre 11, 53, 67–8
exercises: adaptation and habituation 77–8, 94; games 62, 94; relaxation 79

105

Overcoming Common Problems Series

Selected titles

A full list of titles is available from Sheldon Press,
36 Causton Street, London SW1P 4ST and on our website at
www.sheldonpress.co.uk

The A to Z of Eating Disorders
Emma Woolf

Autism and Asperger Syndrome in Adults
Dr Luke Beardon

Chronic Pain the Drug-free Way
Phil Sizer

Coping Successfully with Hiatus Hernia
Dr Tom Smith

Coping with Aggressive Behaviour
Dr Jane McGregor

Coping with Diverticulitis
Peter Cartwright

Coping with Headaches and Migraine
Alison Frith

Coping with Memory Problems
Dr Sallie Baxendale

Coping with the Psychological Effects of Illness
Dr Fran Smith, Dr Carina Eriksen
and Professor Robert Bor

Dementia Care: A guide
Christina Macdonald

Depression and Anxiety the Drug-free Way
Mark Greener

Depressive Illness: The curse of the strong
Dr Tim Cantopher

Dr Dawn's Guide to Sexual Health
Dr Dawn Harper

Dr Dawn's Guide to Toddler Health
Dr Dawn Harper

Dr Dawn's Guide to Your Baby's First Year
Dr Dawn Harper

Dying for a Drink: All you need to know to beat the booze
Dr Tim Cantopher

The Empathy Trap: Understanding antisocial personalities
Dr Jane McGregor and Tim McGregor

Everything Your GP Doesn't Have Time to Tell You about Arthritis
Dr Matt Piccaver

Gestational Diabetes: Your survival guide to diabetes in pregnancy
Dr Paul Grant

The Heart Attack Survival Guide
Mark Greener

The Holistic Guide for Cancer Survivors
Mark Greener

How to Stop Worrying
Dr Frank Tallis

IBS: Dietary advice to calm your gut
Alex Gazzola and Julie Thompson

Living with Angina
Dr Tom Smith

Living with Multiple Sclerosis
Mark Greener

Living with Tinnitus and Hyperacusis
Dr Laurence McKenna, Dr David Baguley
and Dr Don McFerran

Mental Health in Children and Young People: Spotting symptoms and seeking help early
Dr Sarah Vohra

The Multiple Sclerosis Diet Book
Tessa Buckley

Overcoming Gambling: A guide for problem and compulsive gamblers
Philip Mawer

Parenting Your Disabled Child: The first three years
Margaret Barrett

Sleep Better: The science and the myths
Professor Graham Law and Dr Shane Pascoe

Stress-related Illness
Dr Tim Cantopher

Taming the Beast Within: Understanding personality disorder
Professor Peter Tyrer

Therapy Pets: A guide
Jill Eckersley

Toxic People: Dealing with dysfunctional relationships
Dr Tim Cantopher

Treating Arthritis: The drug-free way
Margaret Hills and Christine Horner

Treating Arthritis Diet Book
Margaret Hills

Understanding Hoarding
Jo Cooke

Vertigo and Dizziness
Jaydip Ray

Your Guide for the Cancer Journey: Cancer and its treatment
Mark Greener

Lists of titles in the Mindful Way and Sheldon Short Guides series are also available from Sheldon Press.